Know-It-All
Medicine

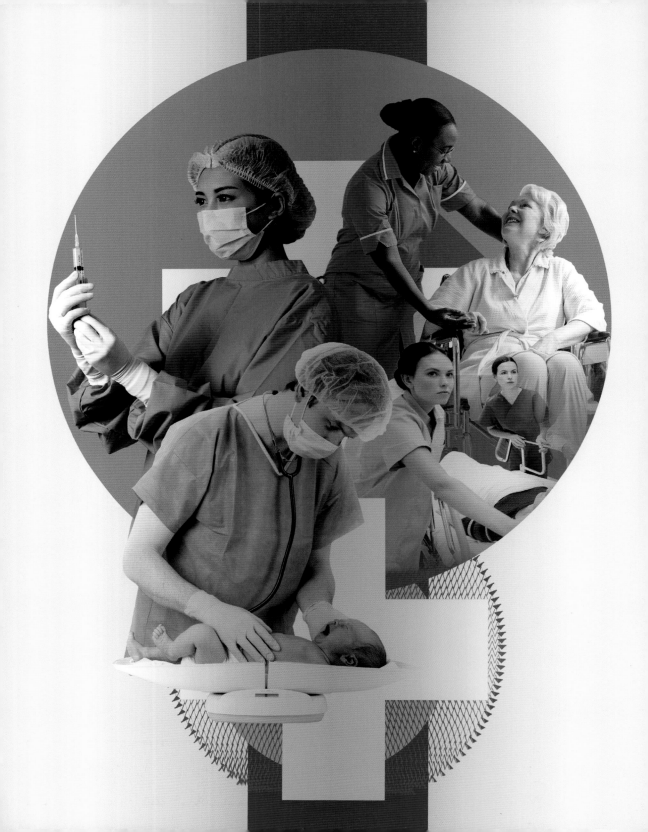

Know-It-All
Medicine

The 50 Crucial Milestones, Treatments & Technologies in the History of Health, Each Explained in Under a Minute >

Editor **Dr. Gabrielle M. Finn**

Contributors
Philip Cox
Dr. Gabrielle M. Finn
Laura Fitton
Joanna Matthan
Larissa Nelson
Martin Veysey

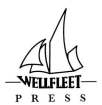

WELLFLEET
P R E S S

Quarto is the authority on a wide range of topics.

Quarto educates, entertains and enriches the lives of our readers—enthusiasts and lovers of hands-on living.

www.quartoknows.com

First published in the United States of America in 2017 by Wellfleet Press, a member of Quarto Publishing Group USA Inc.
142 West 36th Street, 4th Floor
New York, New York 10018
www.QuartoKnows.com

10 9 8 7 6 5 4 3 2 1

ISBN: 978-1-57715-149-4

This book was conceived, designed, and produced by

Ivy Press
An imprint of The Quarto Group
The Old Brewery, 6 Blundell Street
London N7 9BH, United Kingdom
T (0)20 7700 6700 F (0)20 7700 8066

Publisher **Susan Kelly**
Creative Director **Michael Whitehead**
Editorial Director **Tom Kitch**
Commissioning Editor **Sophie Collins**
Senior Project Editor **Caroline Earle**
Designer **Ginny Zeal**
Picture Researcher **Katie Greenwood**
Illustrator **Steve Rawlings**
Glossaries Text **Gabrielle M. Finn**

Printed in China

CONTENTS

INTRODUCTION
Dr. Gabrielle M. Finn

Medicine is the science of the diagnosis, treatment, and prevention of disease. Its history is steeped in gore, antiquity, and pioneering discovery from the rituals of early medicine and the musings of Leonardo da Vinci, to modern-day advances in cloning and bionics. This book is aimed at presenting some of the most interesting topics in medicine as easy-to-swallow pills that won't stick in the throat of the reader. We'll explore some of the early providers of medical care, such as shamans and witch doctors and end with pioneering advancements, including artificial limbs and laboratory-grown organs.

How medicine is encountered by individuals is determined by their culture and health status—whether it be homeopathy and Chinese traditional medicines or radiotherapy and surgery. That said, the language of medicine is commonplace in everyday culture. Diseases and drugs are accepted sites on the biological landscape. Although many of us have well-stocked medicine cabinets in our bathrooms, frequently we don't truly understand the ailment nor the true purpose of the pill we are about to reach for. This is something we hope to change once you have read this book.

Medicine has evolved at a phenomenal rate—the technologies and treatments now utilized on a daily basis, such as dialysis and radiotherapy, would not so long ago have been regarded as the content of a science fiction movie. Imagine where medicine could be within the next decade or century. If we can engineer bionic limbs and conduct surgery using robots now—what is next?

Without using technical language, we will demystify a range of treatments including cochlear implants to restore hearing, bionic limbs controlled by the patient, and organ donation. You'll become an expert on imaging, from X-rays to MRI, ultrasound to CT scans, and we'll tell you all you need to know about treatments such as chemotherapy and preventative medicine, including vaccinations and contraception.

The observations of the ancient Greek physician Hippocrates laid the foundations of modern medicine.

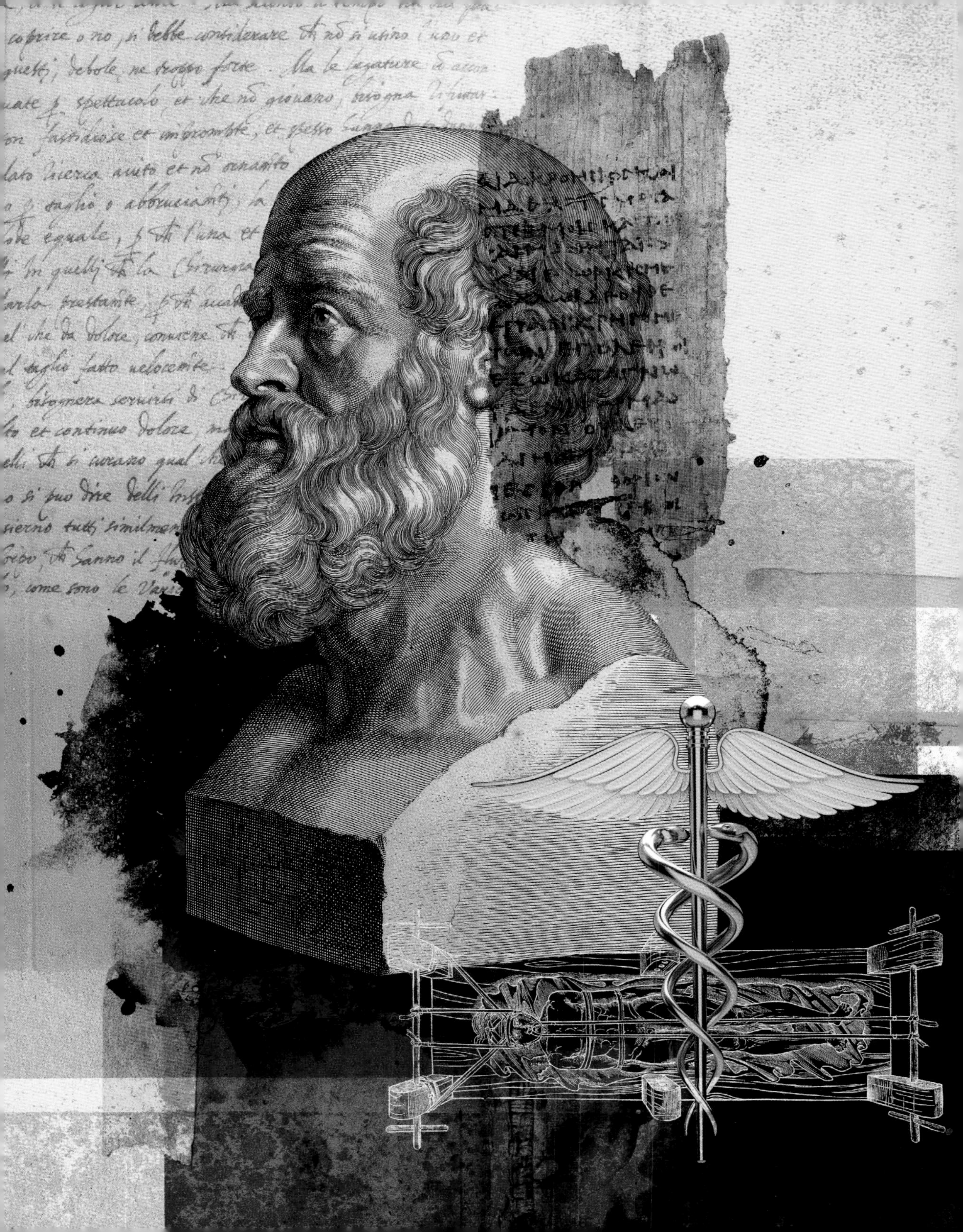

Medicine is a fascinating yet complex subject. It covers a plethora of topics including the anatomy of the body, surgery, therapies, treatments, drugs, and diseases, to name but a few. To chronicle the history of medicine within one book would be quite a feat; instead, I have chosen topics that demonstrate the origins of medicine, milestones in treatments, and explain some of the most commonly encountered diseases and treatments.

How This Book Works

This book won't answer your every question but it is hoped that it will spark your interest to read further. Its structure is simple—you can start anywhere. Fifty topics are presented, each is succinct and can be read in isolation, or you may wish to read a chapter at a time. The topics present a quick overview in the "3-second dose," the bulk of the topic is covered in the succinct main entry followed by additional interesting information within the "3-minute treatment."

A team of scientists and medics have crafted a journey for you through medical history avoiding jargon and presenting a concise crash course. Our journey starts with **Early & Non-Traditional Medicine** where we consider the roots of medicine in folklore and ancient traditions. Moving forward we consider **Landmark Advances** where we explore some of the biggest and most renowned advances in medical history. Within **Imaging & Technology** we look at the mechanisms available to sneak a peek below the surface of the body to discover what lurks beneath. Once we have used imaging to discover the mechanics, we move on to explore the array of **Treatments, Therapies & Procedures** available to patients. Within the chapter on **Diseases** we discover how different conditions present and their associated symptoms, treatments, and prognoses. The medical team is ever expanding, and within the **Roles in Medicine** chapter we learn about the responsibilities of key members of a medical team that a patient would commonly encounter. Our journey terminates with **Drugs** where we study how a range of drugs work, from those in the bathroom cabinet to some with a little more notoriety. Interspersed within each chapter are biographical profiles of some eminent figures from medicine, each with a timeline of their lives and achievements.

Landmark advances such as Alexander Fleming's discovery of antibiotics revolutionized the treatment of bacterial infections.

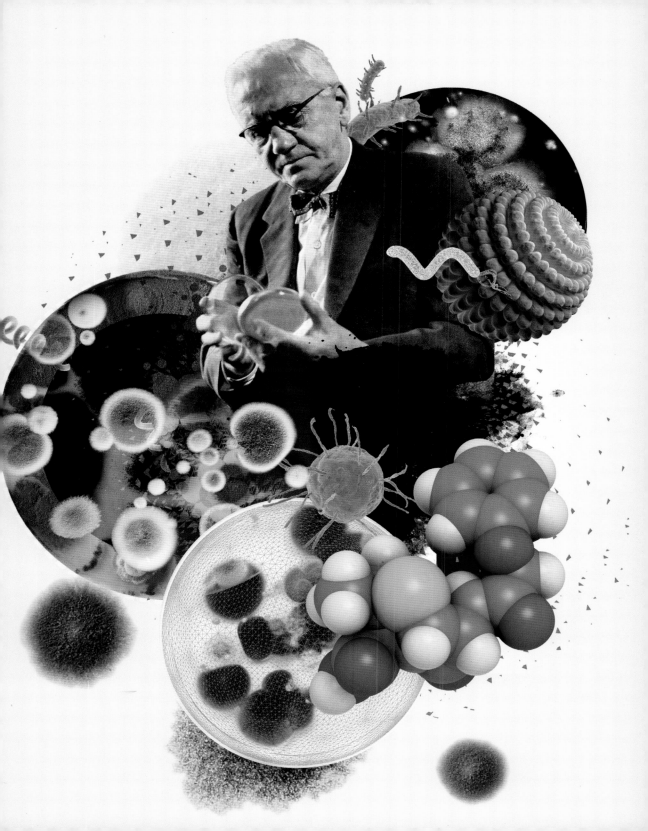

EARLY & NON-TRADITIONAL MEDICINE

EARLY & NON-TRADITIONAL MEDICINE
GLOSSARY

acupuncture A technique derived from ancient Chinese medicine, acupuncture involves the insertion of fine needles into specific sites in the body for therapeutic or preventative purposes. It is classed as an alternative form of medicine.

alternative medicine A term used to describe treatments and procedures that fall outside the routine methods used within mainstream healthcare. Examples include homeopathy, osteopathy, and acupuncture.

Asklepion An ancient Greek hospital, dedicated to the god of health, Asklepios. It was built in 357 BCE near Kos in Greece.

Ayurvedic medicine Considered to be the world's oldest healthcare system. It evolved in India and is holistic. Ayurvedic medicine strives to create harmony between the body, mind, and spirit, because it is thought that such balance prevents illness and prolongs life.

blood-letting The withdrawal of blood from a patient to cure or prevent illness and disease. It is an ancient practice but still occurs today in some cultures.

family doctor Family doctors, also known as family physicians, are doctors who provide primary and continuing medical care for patients in the community. Family doctors treat some illnesses but can also refer patients to hospital clinics for further assessment or treatment.

herbal remedy Plant extracts that may be eaten or applied to the skin in order to treat a medical condition or assist the function of the body. They have been used medicinally since ancient times.

Hippocratic Oath An oath historically taken by doctors. It was written by Hippocrates and is one of the most widely known of Greek medical texts. The oath required a new doctor to swear by a number of healing gods and to uphold ethical standards. Similar versions still exist today.

holistic medicine A healthcare system that focuses on looking at the whole person. It includes consideration of physical, nutritional, environmental, emotional, social, spiritual, and lifestyle factors.

magico-religious Having the character of a body of magical practices intended to cause a supernatural being to produce or prevent a specific result. Some religions have elements of magico-religious beliefs that allow followers to use magic to enable divine intervention in human affairs.

pseudoscience Something that claims to be scientific but that does not adhere to a specific scientific method.

purging The act of ridding something within the body such as food, toxins, an unwanted feeling, memory, or condition.

quackery The promotion of fraudulent, unsafe, or ignorant medical practices.

succussion The process of shaking violently. In homeopathy, succussion refers to the series of dilutions and strikings required to prepare the medication. Within medicine it specifically refers to a method of shaking to detect the presence of fluid and air in a body cavity.

welfare state The role of a government in both the protection and promotion of the economic and social well-being of its citizens. It can comprise expenditures that are intended to improve health, education, employment, and social security.

SHAMANS & WITCH DOCTORS

RELATED ENTRIES
See also
ORIGINS OF MEDICINE
page 16

HOMEOPATHY
page 20

TRADITIONAL
CHINESE MEDICINE
page 24

3-SECOND DOSE
Shamans achieved religious ecstasy in ritualistic ceremonies and hobnobbed with spirits to placate them to restore health, whereas witch doctors had access to protective remedies against witchcraft.

3-MINUTE TREATMENT
Shamans' and witch doctors' magico-religious ritualism to cure illness makes them the most influential healers of premodern society. Although not similar to modern medicine, their doctoring is used as the base point for measuring the progress of medicine through the ages. Some branches of modern medicine can be traced back to these prehistoric roots and have included ritualized or symbolic elements of tribal or indigenous medicine to drive away sickness by accessing the mind.

Premodern healers helped the unwell in society make sense of sickness at a time when medicine as a cure for disease was not part of the common experience. The shamans of old were possessors of magico-religious powers and were versed in the ancient traditions of indigenous societies. As healers, they were indispensable in all ceremonies involving the human soul, as disease was associated with the soul either straying away or having been stolen by a benevolent or malevolent spirit of the recently dead. The mainstay of their treatment was to locate the soul via a trance-like state, recapture it and coax it to return to the body, thus restoring well-being. Witch doctors were highly revered folk healers in tribal societies with the ability to heal those with conditions caused specifically by witchcraft. Their magical powers of divination and healing, and their access to the spirits of benevolent ancestors, meant they were able to counter powerful witchcraft—the usual suspect for all illness. In Europe, witch doctors came to be synonymous with quackery, imposters associated with conning the ill and infirm using superstition or suspicious forms of medication for personal gain. Today, rather derogatorily, practitioners of alternative medicine, such as faith healers, are sometimes referred to under this umbrella term.

3-SECOND BIOGRAPHY
W. H. R. RIVERS
1864–1922
English neurologist, psychologist, ethnologist, and anthropologist who paved the way for research into prehistoric doctoring and native medical practices

EXPERT
Joanna Matthan

Before the development of modern medicine, healers used various magico-religious rituals and ceremonies to cure the sick.

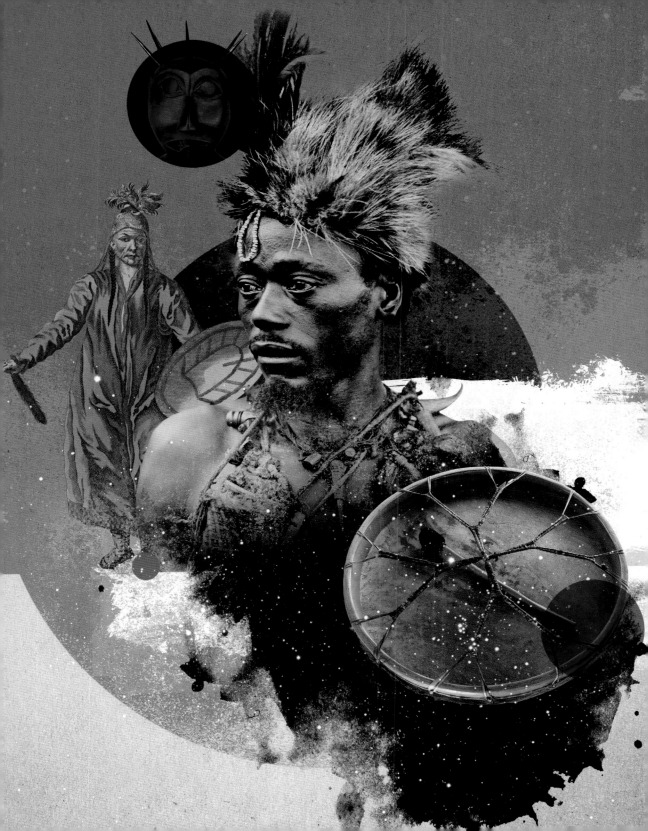

ORIGINS OF MEDICINE

3-SECOND DOSE
Barber-surgeons, body-snatchers, and early anatomical studies were linked together by the laws of supply and demand.

3-MINUTE TREATMENT
Human dissections were common in ancient Egypt and Greece. Early modern anatomical studies began in Italy: anatomists in Bologna dissected cadavers to understand the workings of internal organs. Medicine had become a truly scientific profession. Body-snatchers are sometimes, mistakenly, called graverobbers. Graverobbers, however, stuck to thieving valuables from tombs and from the dead. Some body-snatchers, notably Burke and Hare in the 1800s in Edinburgh, resorted to murdering people instead of simply stealing dead bodies.

Barber-surgeons performed operations on the war-wounded all over medieval Europe. Their other daily tasks included cutting hair and blood-letting, extracting teeth, selling (questionable) medicines, and administering enemas. These were not educated men—many could not even read; they learned their trade by being apprenticed to someone more experienced. Surgeons started to be university educated in the 1700s. As surgeons attempted to become respectable professionals, anatomical studies increased in importance in European medicine. By dissecting bodies and learning from them, doctors distanced themselves from professions they associated with quackery (botanical studies and homeopathy). More and more cadavers were required to teach students, and this increased demand led to the start of the illegal trade of body-snatching. At night, body-snatchers slipped into graveyards, dug up the recently dead and supplied them to the ready hands of dissectors. They did not need to fear a prison sentence as long as they were not tempted into stealing the belongings of the dead. Before the 1830s, only those condemned to "death and dissection" were available legally; the bodies of unclaimed individuals (usually workhouse dwellers) could also be used. Dissecting had to be done quickly to avoid the stench of putrefying bodies.

RELATED ENTRIES
See also
HIPPOCRATES
page 18

HOMEOPATHY
page 20

JOSEPH LISTER
page 38

ANESTHESIA & SURGERY
page 80

3-SECOND BIOGRAPHIES
AMBROISE PARÉ
1510–90
French barber-surgeon whose work raised the professional status of surgery

ANDREAS VESALIUS
1514–64
Flemish anatomist who produced a monumental atlas of human anatomy, *De human corpori fabrica* (1543), which was the start of experimental approaches to understand medicine

EXPERT
Joanna Matthan

As surgery became a profession, demand for bodies to dissect and study increased.

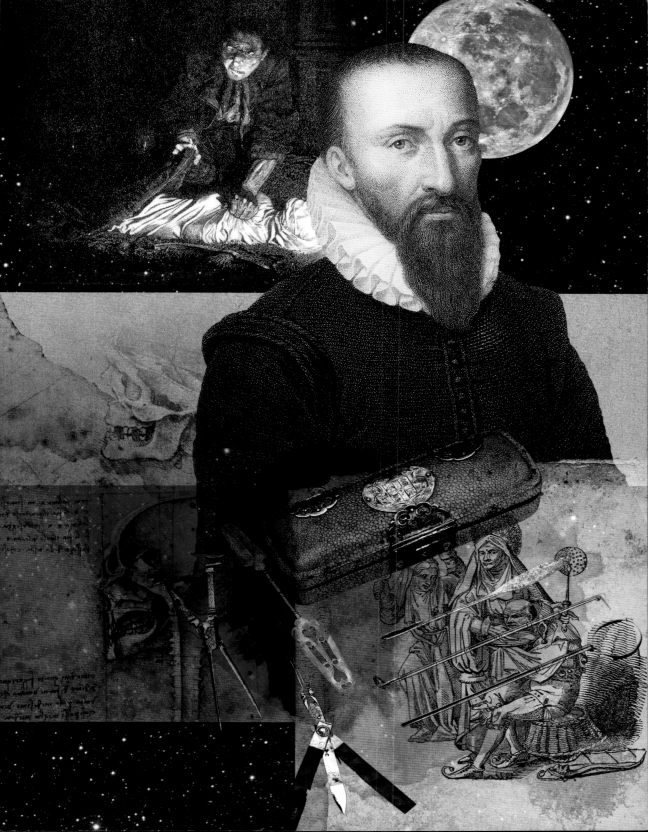

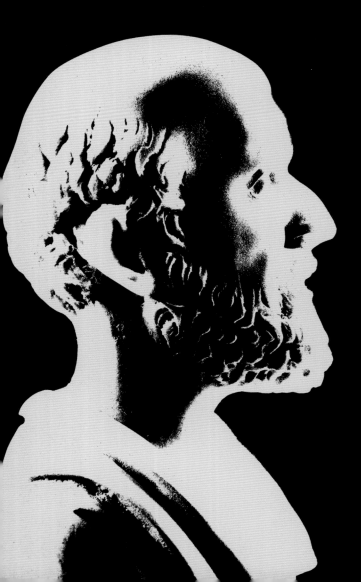

c. 460 BCE
Born on the Greek island of Kos, the son of Heracleides (a physician) and Praxithea

c. 455–435 BCE
Receives nine years of formative schooling, followed by two years of secondary school and a medical apprenticeship; undertakes formal medical training at the Asklepion (healing temple) of Kos

430–427 BCE
Spends three years in Athens, plague-ridden at the time; thought to have cured the King of Macedonia of tuberculosis

431–404 BCE
Peloponnesian War: the height of Hippocrates' career

400 BCE
Founds School of Medicine in Kos and combines his teaching and doctoring roles; likely to have apprenticed his sons, Draco and Thessalus, and his son-in-law, Polybus, to medicine

c. 370 BCE (earliest 374 BCE, latest 350 BCE)
Dies in Larissa, Thessaly

HIPPOCRATES

Medicine owes a huge debt of thanks to the "Father of Western Medicine," the classical Greek doctor, Hippocrates (of Kos), for his radically different way of looking at the relationship between the causes of sickness and the treatment of disease, and for founding the Hippocratic School of Medicine, where observation and objective documentation were emphasized—these would become the basis of modern medicine. Medicine became a profession distinct from any other as a result of his efforts. Previously, physicians had blamed disease on anything from the position of the stars to the discontent of the gods. Hippocrates insisted that reason should guide the diagnosis and treatment of illness. He observed patients and used these observations and his experience to make a diagnosis, to treat, and also to give an estimate of how the disease would progress (prognosis).

Not much is known about Hippocrates' private life. Most is likely to be legend or to have been embellished over time. Even his birth and death dates are circumspect. He was born around 460 BCE on the Greek island of Kos to a wealthy family. His father and grandfather were doctors, so Hippocrates probably received the best possible education and was then apprenticed to his relatives. He received his formal medical training at the Asklepion of Kos, but also took lessons from another physician, Herodicus. He is known to have traveled widely, to have fathered two sons and a daughter, doctored to the needs of the high and mighty (he is said to have cured the King of Macedonia of tuberculosis), and spent at least three years in plague-ridden Athens.

Hippocrates and his followers described numerous medical conditions. Hippocratic fingers, today called finger clubbing, commonly seen in a certain type of heart or lung disease, was first described by him. Modern medicine can thank him for instilling discipline, rigorous practice, and strict professionalism into the code of conduct for doctors. A Hippocratic physician would seek to be honest, calm, serious, understanding, and well-kept at all times. Doctors around the world still take the Hippocratic Oath when they graduate, but in a newer and more culturally appropriate form.

Hippocrates is also considered to be the author of the *Hippocratic Corpus*, a collection of around 60 to 70 medically related works, but it is more likely that this monumental collection was penned by a variety of hands. His precise year of death in Larissa is not known but he is thought to have lived into his eighties—perhaps past the 100-year mark.

Joanna Matthan

HOMEOPATHY

RELATED ENTRY
See also
SHAMANS & WITCH DOCTORS
page 14

3-SECOND DOSE
Homeopathy aims to treat illness with highly diluted substances that would, in large doses, produce the illness symptoms in a healthy person.

3-MINUTE TREATMENT
Homeopathy gained in popularity at a time when blood-letting, purging, and other dubious treatments were the main cure for disease and illness. Hahnemann was disgusted by the unscientific treatments he was supposed to apply to his patients and believed that more harm than good was done to his patients using these methods. Thus the simple and less harmful practice of homeopathy came as a welcome relief to many patients and also to some doctors.

Homeopathy was widely used throughout the nineteenth century as an alternative therapy. It was founded on the principle that "like cures like." In 1796, a German doctor, Samuel Hahnemann, consumed a large dose of quinine (the bark of a Peruvian tree), a popular treatment for malaria, and noticed that his symptoms were similar to those in malaria patients, despite him being well. He experimented with different common treatments and concluded that all diseases could be best treated by those drugs that produced, in healthy people, similar symptoms to those with the disease. Because homeopathy is based on the belief that a small amount of a substance will cure the same symptoms that it causes in large amounts, and that large doses can make a disease worse, the substance is diluted until no molecules can be detected and is vigorously shaken, a process known as succussion. The effect of the medicine is thought to be far more potent the more it is diluted, therefore very small doses are used. No medication is given until other aspects of the patient are considered, such as personality, mental and physical state, and life history. Modern medical science takes a strong stance against systems such as homeopathy and term them pseudosciences, but it remains popular worldwide.

3-SECOND BIOGRAPHIES
HIPPOCRATES
c. 460–c. 377 BCE
Greek doctor and philosopher who may have experimented with homeopathy by treating mania with a small dose of mandrake root, knowing that a larger dose caused mania

PARACELSUS
1493–1541
Swiss alchemist, physician, astrologer, and philosopher who said that a small dose of "what makes a man ill also cures him"

SAMUEL HAHNEMANN
1755–1843
German physician who founded the system of homeopathy

EXPERT
Joanna Matthan

Samuel Hahnemann's experiments led him to the conclusion that "like cures like."

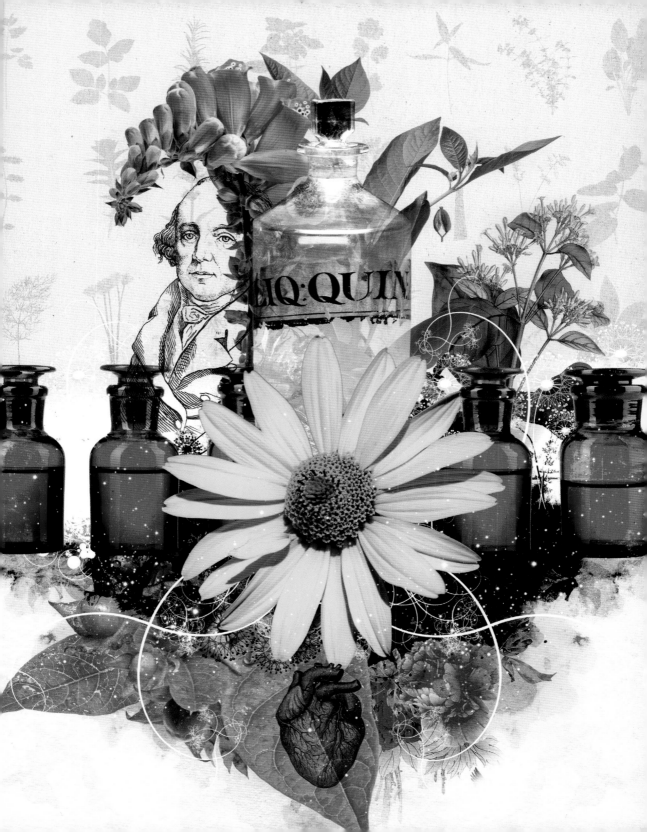

HEALTHCARE SYSTEMS

3-SECOND DOSE
Most countries have some form of healthcare system in place (depending on politics, economy, history) to care for those in society needing medical care.

3-MINUTE TREATMENT
Access to medical care was largely means-based in earlier times. Germany started the first welfare state in the late 1800s. In the UK, the National Health Service was started in 1948 with free healthcare for all. Still, even today, over 400 million people worldwide lack access to essential health services. The 1948 WHO Constitution declared health as a fundamental human right and access to health services is still a high priority for WHO.

Good healthcare systems deliver high-quality services to patients whenever and wherever they need them. These services require a stable financing mechanism, trained and adequately paid healthcare professionals, well-maintained facilities, and the ability to deliver medical care, medicines, and technologies. In entrepreneurial systems, for example the USA, private insurance is for those who can afford it and free state-run hospitals for those who cannot. In socialist countries like Cuba and China, all healthcare provision is by the state. Some countries have a welfare-oriented system, a combination of private contribution and public funding to ensure the less healthy are paid for from a common pool. Others, including the UK and Israel, have comprehensive universal care for all (although private systems also exist). Healthcare is generally provided by a tier system. Primary care services are usually the first point-of-call for patients and are provided by family doctors who have a wide breadth of knowledge. Secondary care is the next step for ailments that require specialist knowledge and is generally accessed via referrals from primary care. Tertiary care is for already hospitalized patients who need an even higher level of specialist care. These are usually larger medical centers with specialized equipment and expert knowledge.

3-SECOND BIOGRAPHIES
OTTO VON BISMARCK
1815–98
German 1st chancellor and politician who implemented the world's first welfare state in the 1880s and in 1883 set up state-run medical insurance (Sickness Insurance Law)

WILLIAM BEVERIDGE
1879–1963
British economist and social reformer who published the Beveridge Report in 1942 recommending the government find ways to fight "Want, Disease, Ignorance, Squalor, and Idleness"; the National Health Service was started in 1948 based on his recommendations

EXPERT
Joanna Matthan

Although their funding mechanisms vary around the world, most healthcare systems utilize a structure of primary, secondary, and tertiary treatment.

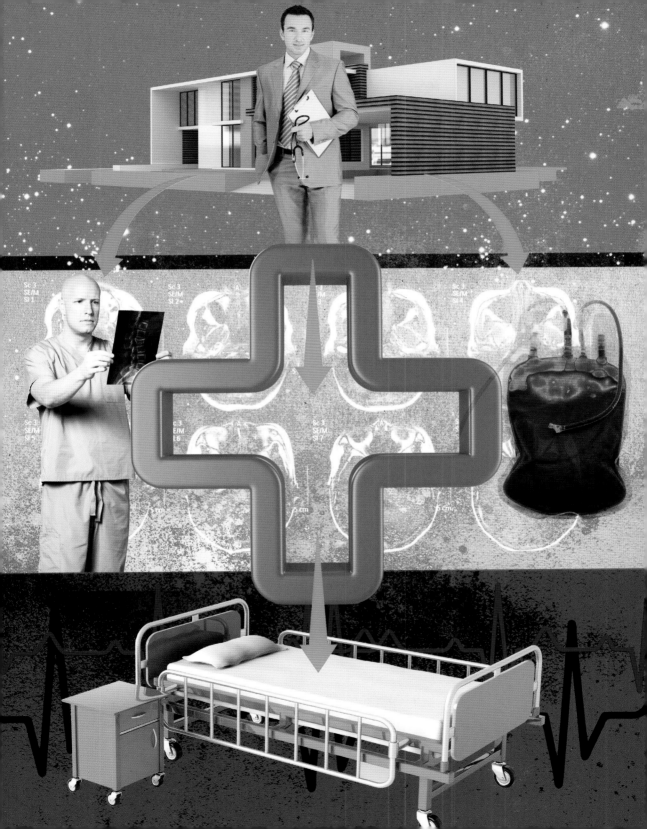

TRADITIONAL CHINESE MEDICINE (TCM)

Traditional Chinese Medicine

has its roots in an age-old medical system that aims to either prevent or heal illness by retaining or restoring a person's natural yin-yang balance. It includes a wide variety of alternative medical practices, from acupuncture and herbal remedies to dietary therapy, massage, and exercise, and it is widely used in China and in the West. TCM is based on the firm belief that the body is a representation of a microcosm of nature and society (similar to Hippocratic medicine). Qi is the vital energy that permeates the body, circulating through meridians (channels connecting organs). In living beings, life arises from build-up of qi—and death is dissipation of qi. TCM healers aim to restore the distribution of qi by balancing yin (passive, interior) and yang (active, exterior), the two dynamic forces that are present in the human body and in the universe. When there is harmony between these two cyclical forces, one is healthy. Breakdown of equilibrium between yin and yang results in illness. A key part of TCM is acupuncture, where thin needles are introduced into the body at known acupuncture points to relieve pain and treat other conditions. This is the most widely used TCM practice worldwide. Because of the lack of evidence on its effectiveness, the scientific world considers TCM a pseudoscience.

3-SECOND DOSE
TCM is a system of healing that follows an ancient healing tradition and includes balancing yin and yang forces through herbal remedies and acupuncture.

3-MINUTE TREATMENT
TCM is considered to represent unadulterated holistic ancient Chinese medicine but it has absorbed countless influences from Indian Ayurvedic medicine and Buddhism and from numerous other regions, combining healing of both mind and soul. Four ancient works (authors unknown) form the classical TCM tradition; the earliest is *The Yellow Emperor's Classic of Internal Medicine*, dating to the third century BCE, and provides TCM's theoretical basis. Chinese herbal remedies and acupuncture date back over 2,200 years.

RELATED ENTRIES
See also
SHAMANS & WITCH DOCTORS
page 14

HIPPOCRATES
page 18

HOMEOPATHY
page 20

3-SECOND BIOGRAPHY
LI SHIZHEN
1518–93
Han Chinese medical doctor, scientist, pharmacologist, herbalist, acupuncturist, and polymath who published the *Compendium of Materia Medica* (*Bencao Gangmu*) in 1578, which lists 1,892 drugs and 11,000 formal prescriptions for different illnesses

EXPERT
Joanna Matthan

Acupuncture seeks to restore the flow of qi by targeting specific points of the body. It is an ancient technique that remains widely popular today.

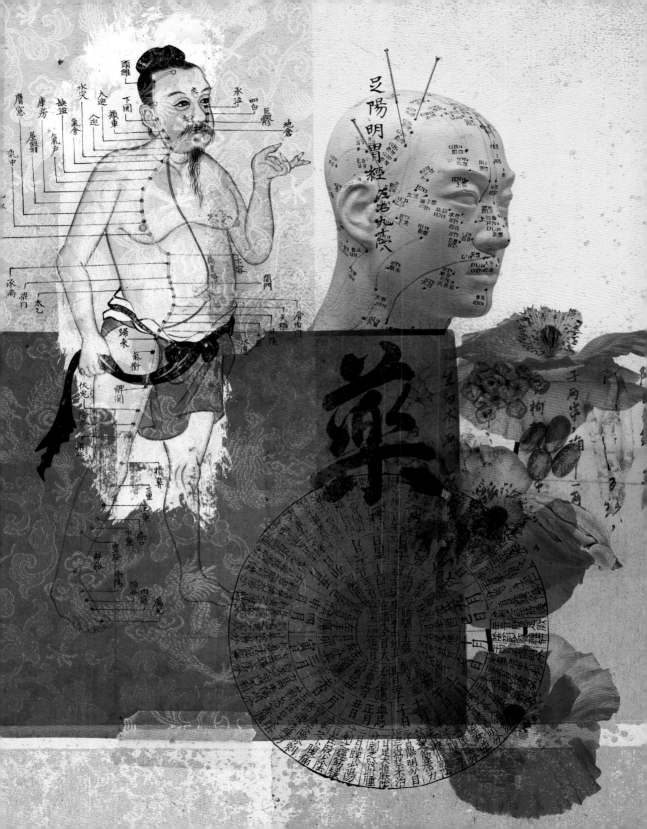

LANDMARK ADVANCES

LANDMARK ADVANCES
GLOSSARY

acute disease A disease with a relatively sudden onset of symptoms that are usually severe.

antiseptic A substance that is applied to living tissue or skin to reduce the possibility of infection.

blood group A blood group, or blood type, is a classification of your blood according to the presence of different substances. There are four main blood groups: A, B, AB, and O. The patient's blood group is determined by the genes they inherited from their parents.

blood vessel A tube that carries blood through the body. There are three types: veins, arteries, and capillaries.

chronic disease Chronic refers to a condition or disease that is persistent or otherwise long-lasting in its effects. Typically chronic diseases are those that last over three months.

congenital A disease or physical abnormality that is present from birth.

DNA Deoxyribonucleic acid (DNA) is a molecule that carries the genetic instructions used in the development, functioning, and reproduction of all known living organisms.

embalming The treatment of an entire or parts of a dead body to protect it from decay. Fixative chemicals are used for this preservation process.

embryo An animal in the early stages of growth. In a human, a baby is an embryo from the time of implantation in the womb until the end of the eighth week after conception.

fetus The embryo of a mammal in the later stages of development, when it shows all the main recognizable features of the mature animal. A human embryo is known as a fetus from the end of the second month of pregnancy until birth.

gene therapy An experimental technique that uses genes to treat or prevent disease. There are three main mechanisms:
1 Replacing a mutated (permanently altered) gene that causes disease with a healthy copy of the gene,
2 Inactivating, or "knocking out," a mutated gene that is malfunctioning, and
3 Introducing a new gene into the body to help fight a disease.

myoelectric A myoelectric signal, also known as a motor action potential, is an electrical impulse that produces contraction of muscle fibers in the body. An example is the skeletal muscles that control voluntary movements.

tendons A robust band of fibrous connective tissue that typically connects muscle to bone. Tendons are capable of withstanding tension from muscle and bone movement.

ultrasound Also known as diagnostic sonography or ultrasonography, ultrasound uses high frequency sound waves to view structures inside the body. It is performed by a practitioner called a sonographer.

vein A blood vessel (tube) forming part of the blood circulation system of the body. It carries mainly deoxygenated blood towards the heart.

ORGAN DONATION & TRANSPLANT

3-SECOND DOSE
A surgical procedure whereby a healthy organ or tissue is transplanted from a living or dead individual—the donor—to a recipient who is need of a transplant.

3-MINUTE TREATMENT
Organ donation differs from body donation, where a person donates their entire body to a medical school for research and teaching purposes. This process involves embalming the body and no tissues are used in live recipients. Bodies that are donated are used for dissection and rehearsal or surgical procedures. This process is highly governed by laws in each country.

Donated organs are given to patients who have damaged or diseased organs. The transplanted organ can cure them or significantly improve their condition. Organs can be transplanted from living donors, brain-dead donors, or from the deceased (cadaveric) donors, provided organs are harvested within a short time frame. Organs that are frequently transplanted include the heart, kidneys, liver, lungs, pancreas, intestine, and thymus. It is increasingly common for other tissues such as cornea, skin, bones, tendons, heart valves, nerves, and blood vessels to be transplanted. The kidneys are the most frequently transplanted organ worldwide. Organ and tissue donation relies on genetic matches between donor and recipient. Without compatible blood groups, the tissue will be rejected by the recipient's body. The need for a compatible match creates long waiting lists, and often patients die as a result of organ failure before a suitable donor can be found. With organs such as the liver, where part of it can be harvested, or paired organs such as the kidneys, where someone can function with only one, it is common for family members to donate organs to ill relatives. Living donations are well planned. Donations from the deceased, however, are opportunistic so the process must be fast and highly organized—tissue can die within six hours.

RELATED ENTRIES
See also
BIONIC ORGANS
page 42

3-D PRINTING & BIOPRINTING
page 64

3-SECOND BIOGRAPHY
JOSEPH EDWARD MURRAY
1919–2012
American surgeon who conducted the first successful kidney transplant; in 1990, he was awarded the Nobel Prize in Physiology or Medicine

EXPERT
Gabrielle M. Finn

Organ transplants are highly organized operations and, in the case of donations from cadavers, speed is of the essence.

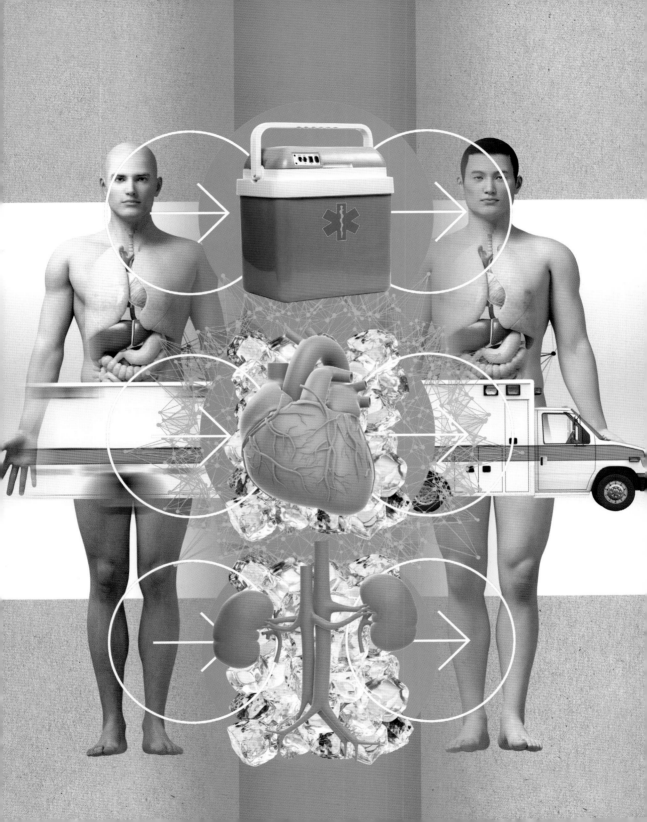

IN VITRO FERTILIZATION (IVF)

3-SECOND DOSE

IVF is a process where an egg is fertilized by a sperm outside of the human body in vitro ("in glass").

3-MINUTE TREATMENT

Conventional IVF exposes the egg to multiple sperm in a dish but no direct sperm injection takes place. IVF is often confused with Intra-Cytoplasmic Sperm Injection (ICSI). IVF and ICSI both involve fertilization outside the body; however, during ICSI a single sperm is injected into part of the egg known as the cytoplasm. ICSI is used when sperm are immobile or misshapen.

IVF is a treatment used to enable people with fertility issues to conceive a child. Babies born following IVF are often referred to as "test-tube babies" as their creation takes place within a laboratory, inside glass dishes. IVF requires eggs to be collected from the ovaries, conducted in theater with ultrasound guidance, usually after a course of drugs to stimulate the ovary to produce multiple eggs. The eggs are then introduced to sperm in a glass dish. The sperm then compete to fertilize the egg. Only one sperm is needed to fertilize the egg, and if this is successful an embryo is formed. The embryo is allowed to grow in the lab, where optimal conditions are ensured, for a few days. The amount of time depends on the quality of the embryo. The embryo is then transferred back to the woman's uterus (or the uterus of a surrogate) using a small tube (catheter) inserted into the vagina. Drugs (hormones) are given to promote the embryo to implant into the lining of the uterus (endometrium) and develop into a baby. In some cases more than one embryo is implanted, which can lead to multiple births. Legislation in some countries allows same-sex couples or single people to use IVF or ICSI for conception. In either case, sperm or egg donation can be used. Surrogates can also be used to carry the developing baby.

RELATED ENTRIES

See also
ULTRASOUND
page 56

CONTRACEPTION
page 74

3-SECOND BIOGRAPHIES

ROBERT EDWARDS
1925–2013
British physiologist who pioneered IVF; in 2010 he was awarded a Nobel Prize for his work

ROBERT WINSTON
1940–
British professor of fertility and a gynecologist responsible for many advances in IVF, specifically genetic screening of embryos

LOUISE BROWN
1978–
The first "test-tube baby" following IVF; she was born via Caesarean section in Oldham, UK

EXPERT
Gabrielle M. Finn

IVF can help infertile and same-sex couples to conceive.

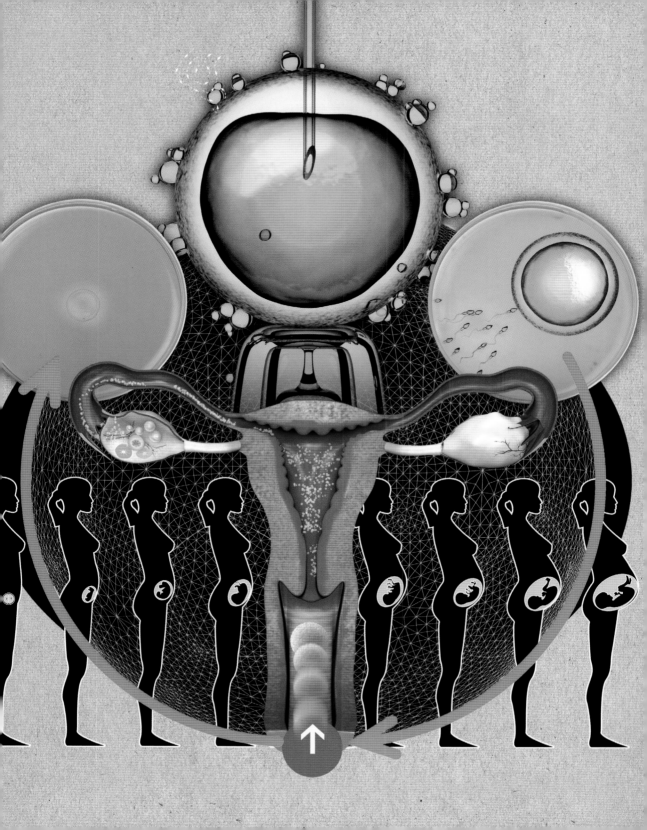

BYPASS & PACEMAKERS

3-SECOND DOSE

In motoring, a bypass is a road that provides an alternative route—in medicine, a coronary bypass circumvents blocked vessels to improve blood flow.

3-MINUTE TREATMENT

Gastric bypass is becoming increasingly common. It involves surgically bypassing the stomach and making it smaller as a way to tackle obesity. A section of stomach is stapled to make it smaller and attached directly to part of the small intestine, bypassing the main, larger part of the stomach. Patients whose stomachs have been bypassed are unable to eat as much food and will feel full quicker and for longer.

Many procedures for treating

heart problems have been pioneered over the decades. One of the most common now used is the coronary artery bypass graft, a surgical procedure used to treat coronary heart disease. This involves removing a vessel from elsewhere in the patient's body, usually the saphenous vein in the leg, and surgically grafting it to provide an alternative route for blood flow—this bypasses the vessels that have been blocked by heart disease. The surgery lasts around six hours, and involves the surgeons breaking the breastbone (sternum) to access the heart. Sometimes more than one graft is required if multiple vessels are blocked, for example a triple heart bypass. A major advancement in medical technology was the invention of the implantable cardiac pacemaker. The pacemaker is used to treat abnormal heart rhythms—known as arrhythmia. A pacemaker is a small device that is placed in the patient's chest or, less commonly, abdomen, to help control abnormal heart rhythms. Pacemakers use electrical pulses to initiate the heart to beat at a normal, safe rate. If a pacemaker isn't used, a patient with an arrhythmia may not be able to lead a normal, active life due to fatigue, breathlessness, or fainting. Severe arrhythmias can damage vital organs, cause a loss of consciousness, or even death.

RELATED ENTRIES

See also
BLOOD TRANSFUSION & DONATION
page 82

VASCULAR DISEASE
page 98

ANTICOAGULANTS
page 148

3-SECOND BIOGRAPHY

WILSON GREATBATCH
1919–2011
American inventor and engineer who developed the first implantable cardiac pacemaker

EXPERT

Gabrielle M. Finn

Bypass grafts and implantable pacemakers have revolutionized the treatment of heart disease.

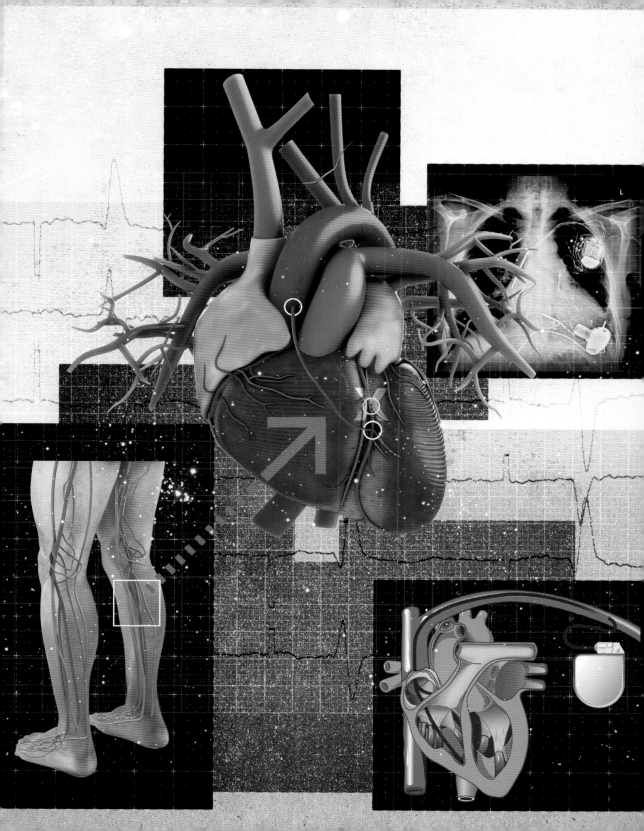

HUMAN GENOME PROJECT (HGP)

RELATED ENTRIES
See also
STEM CELLS & TISSUE
ENGINEERING
page 60

CYSTIC FIBROSIS (CF)
page 108

3-SECOND DOSE
The Human Genome Project mapped out the genome, a human's complete set of deoxyribonucleic acid (DNA) molecules and genes.

3-MINUTE TREATMENT
DNA molecules are made of two paired strands that twist and rotate to form a double helical structure. Each strand is made of four chemical base units, known as nucleotide bases. These are adenine (A), thymine (T), guanine (G), and cytosine (C). Bases on opposite strands in a helix pair specifically—A with T and C with G. The human genome contains around 3 billion nucleotide base pairs. Genes are sections of DNA—each codes for creating a specific protein.

Your genome is the full set of instructions needed to make every cell in your body. The Human Genome Project was a 13-year venture to map the entire human genome. It is considered to be one of the greatest advances in medicine and science. The project relied on the DNA samples of several anonymous volunteers, all from diverse backgrounds. Female DNA samples were derived from blood; males were derived from semen (sperm) samples. The HGP was a worldwide collaboration. The International Human Genome Sequencing Consortium included institutions from the USA, the UK, France, Germany, Japan, and China, where sequencing took place. Over 200 laboratories were involved in mapping the genome. The advantages from this are vast. It provides an understanding of human evolution, genetic diseases, and mutations. The HGP enables improved genetic testing, the creation of new gene therapy treatments and personalized medicines, as well as being able to identify the exact location of genes involved in genetic diseases such as cystic fibrosis. As well as advantages, the HGP has ethical implications. The Ethical, Legal and Social Implications (ELSI) program was established as part of the HGP. Concerns have included the potential for genetic discrimination in employment and health insurance, the integration of genetic testing into medicine, and informed consent.

3-SECOND BIOGRAPHY
CHARLES DELISI
1941–
American professor at Boston University who helped to initiate the Human Genome Project, for which he was awarded the Presidential Citizens Medal by Bill Clinton

EXPERT
Gabrielle M. Finn

The worldwide project to map the human genome—your body's genetic information—was one of the greatest achievements in medical history.

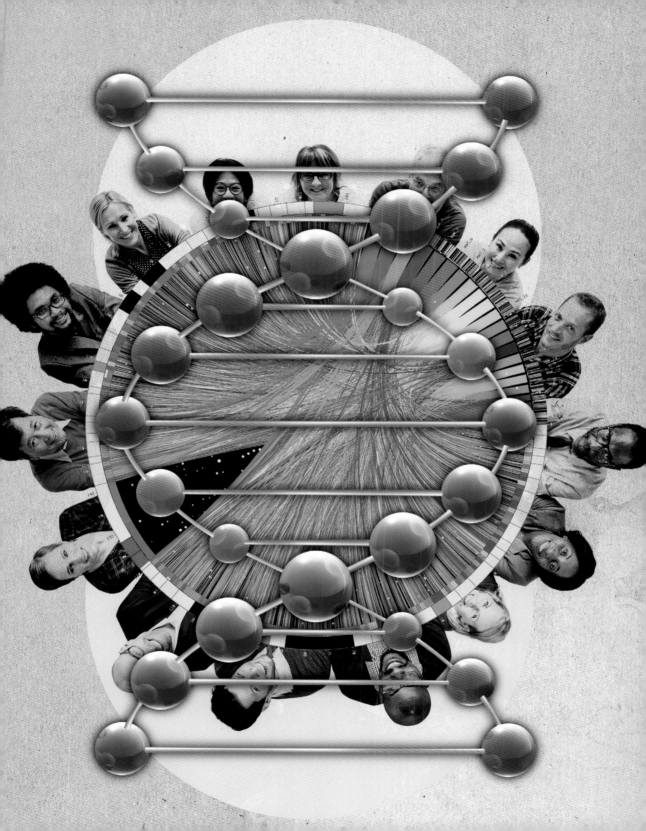

1827
Born in Upton in Essex, England

1838
Attends Grove House School in Tottenham, London

1844
Starts studying medicine at University College London

1852
After graduating from University College London, becomes a Fellow of the Royal College of Surgeons and starts his surgical career in Edinburgh, Scotland

1856
Marries his professor's daughter

1860
Becomes Professor of Surgery at Royal Infirmary in Glasgow, Scotland

1861
Starts working at Glasgow Royal Infirmary, Scotland

1865
Introduces antiseptic (aseptic) surgery

1883
Receives knighthood

1891
Becomes chair of British Institute of Preventive Medicine

1893
Wife dies in Italy during a rare combined holiday, Lister sinks into religious melancholy and loses his lust for life

1896
Retires from a long work life of contributing to science and medicine

1902
Helps save King Edward VII's life by advising on antiseptic surgical methods for an appendectomy (removal of appendix) when no one else wanted to take the responsibility

1912
Dies at his country home in Kent at the age of 84

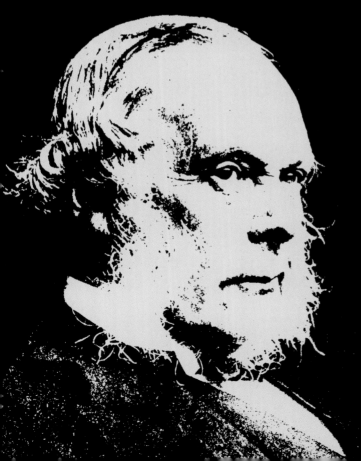

JOSEPH LISTER

Joseph Lister has single-handedly contributed to countless lives being saved. Death, filth, and infection filled the air in operating theaters and hospital wards before Lister's interventions; surgeons' clothes were coated in blood and pus, and hands were generally washed only *after* an operation. Doctors moved between operating theaters, wards, and autopsies (dissections after death) without any attention paid to cleanliness. Lister, a humble and deeply religious English surgeon, could not agree that *sepsis* (from post-surgical wound infections) was just something that happened and he wanted to find an *antisepsis* way of preventing these killer infections.
He had read the French microbiologist Louis Pasteur's germ theory and found it made sense of his own evidence of the spread of infection. He had observed that if patients who had broken bones also had the surrounding skin pierced during the event that caused the injury, this led to a higher death rate from infection. He started washing his hands before operations, wore clean clothes and washed surgical equipment, and dabbed wounds with carbolic acid (the first antiseptic used widely).

Lister was born in Essex and became interested in surgery at an early age. His father, a wealthy wine merchant who was also an inventor, ensured that his son received a broad formal education before he started studying medicine in London. Having successfully completed his studies and, after attaining fellowship of the Royal College of Surgeons, he was recommended to meet James Syme, Professor of Clinical Surgery in Edinburgh. Lister trained under Syme and later married his daughter. He subsequently moved to Glasgow, where he became Professor of Surgery.

Lister's stubbornness in vision and unrelenting experimentation led to his ground-breaking work on antisepsis, infection control, and the introduction of antiseptic surgical techniques. He had to fight against the prevailing belief that post-surgical wound infections somehow magically arose from the wound itself and also against the narrow-mindedness of his colleagues, who ridiculed him at every opportunity. Deaths due to infections after surgery dropped significantly with his methods, and after a period of strong resistance, surgeons adopted his antiseptic techniques.

Known by several titles ("father of modern antisepsis," "father of modern medicine," "father of modern surgery"), Lister's contribution can be seen in countless hospitals worldwide. The food-borne bacteria, *Listeria monocytogenes*, was named after him, and every time you gargle with *Listerine* mouthwash, you are honoring his work in the battle against sepsis.

Joanna Matthan

DIALYSIS

The kidneys are organs in the abdominal cavity that function to remove waste products and excess fluid from the body, ultimately through urine. The process of urine production is required to maintain a stable balance of body chemicals. Patients with chronic kidney disease have a reduced ability to remove waste from the body. If left untreated, the waste products and fluid can build up within the body to dangerously high levels, causing a patient to feel unwell, or even die. Dialysis is used as a treatment to help the body filter out waste and unwanted fluids. There are two main types of dialysis—hemodialysis and peritoneal dialysis. Hemodialysis occurs outside the body and involves a catheter attached to a needle in the patient's arm. Blood travels along the tube into an external dialysis machine for filtration, before being passed back into the arm along another catheter. Sometimes an operation is needed to widen the blood vessels used for the catheter. Hemodialysis occurs a few times a week, usually in hospital. Peritoneal dialysis can be done at the patient's home, often while they sleep. It uses the patient's peritoneum (membrane) to exchange fluids and waste from the blood through a permanent tube, connected to an external dialysis machine.

3-SECOND DOSE

Dialysis is a process of artificially removing waste and unwanted water from the blood—it is used as a treatment for patients whose kidneys don't do this naturally.

3-MINUTE TREATMENT

In an intensive care setting, a patient may undergo hemofiltration. This is similar to dialysis but is driven by convection rather than diffusion. The patient's blood is filtered in a similar manner with replacement fluid added to the blood. Hemofiltration is of greater use for patients with acute kidney injury, sepsis, or multiple organ failure.

RELATED ENTRY

See also
ORGAN DONATION
& TRANSPLANT
page 30

3-SECOND BIOGRAPHY
WILLEM JOHAN KOLFF
1911–2009
Dutch physician who pioneered hemodialysis and artificial organs; he built the first working dialysis machine in 1943 and first successfully treated a patient using hemodialysis in 1945

EXPERT
Gabrielle M. Finn

Dialysis reproduces the waste-removal function normally performed by the kidneys.

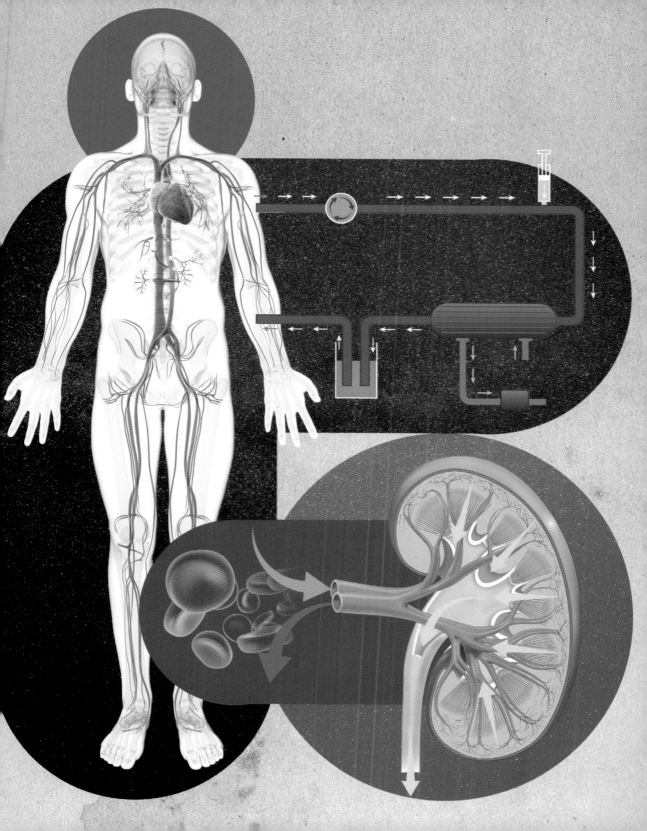

BIONIC ORGANS

Bionic organs are sophisticated feats of engineering that enable the recipient to regain function of missing body parts without the need for careful organ donor matching. Bionics have been used for a number of organs including the heart, pancreas, eyes, and ears. The first bionic hearts were designed in the late 1940s. They were plagued by problems making them more risky than the use of donor organs for transplants. Scientists have worked on the advent of sophisticated bio-prosthetic materials that trick the human immune system into believing the bionic heart is a natural and original part of the body—continued development of these materials could pave the way for major advances. One such advance is the bionic ear. A bionic ear (or cochlear implant) is designed to produce hearing sensations by electrically stimulating nerves inside the ear. It is made up of a number of parts that convert sounds into digital codes. The codes are then converted into electrical impulses and sent along the electrodes positioned in the inner ear (cochlea). The implant's electrodes stimulate the cochlea's nerve, which sends the impulses to the brain where they are interpreted as sound. Scientists have also succeeded in growing miniature, fully functional human kidneys in the lab using skin stem cells—it is hoped these will lead to viable human kidneys for transplantation.

3-SECOND DOSE

Bionic organs are artificial organs that are man-made before being implanted into a patient to replace natural organs that don't function.

3-MINUTE TREATMENT

Scientists are pioneering ways of growing human organs in animal hosts. Techniques currently being investigated include implanting human stem cells into animal embryos or transplanting organs from aborted human fetuses into animal hosts in order to allow the organs to grow to a larger size for transplantation.

RELATED ENTRIES
See also
ORGAN DONATION
& TRANSPLANT
page 30

ARTIFICIAL LIMBS
page 62

3-D PRINTING & BIOPRINTING
page 64

3-SECOND BIOGRAPHIES
GRAEME CLARK
1935–
Australian doctor who pioneered the bionic ear; he is a specialist ear, nose, and throat surgeon

STELIOS ARCADIOU
1946–
Cypriot-Australian performance artist known as Stelarc who grew a third ear on his forearm

EXPERT
Gabrielle M. Finn

Bionic organs can be used instead of human donations. As advances in materials and technology are made, their use could become more widespread.

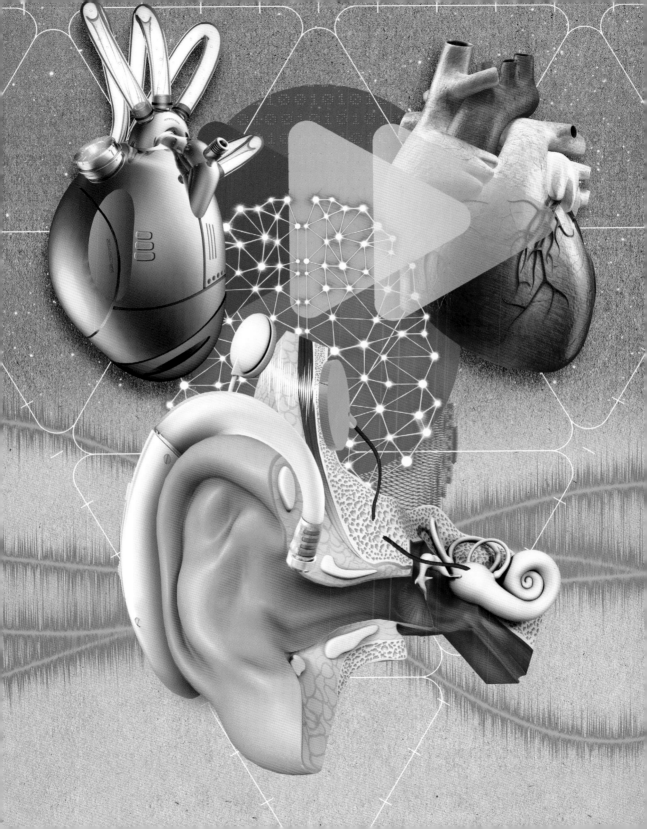

MINIMALLY INVASIVE SURGERY

RELATED ENTRIES
See also
BIONIC ORGANS
page 42

ARTIFICIAL LIMBS
page 62

Minimally invasive surgery is becoming increasingly common as it involves smaller incisions, causes less pain, and usually means faster recovery for patients. Traditional surgery typically utilizes one or two large incisions in order to allow access to the anatomy being operated on. In minimally invasive procedures, however, surgeons make several tiny incisions in the skin. An endoscope (a thin instrument with a miniature camera attached) is passed through one of the incisions. Images from the endoscope are projected onto monitors in the operating theater to enable the underlying anatomy to be visualized and magnified as required. Specially designed instruments are used through the other openings to perform the surgery. In rare cases, a patient may have their surgery changed to traditional surgery during the procedure if the surgeon needs additional access or there is a complication. Organs such as the gall bladder, kidneys, and parts of the liver can all be removed using minimally invasive procedures. Although minimally invasive surgery can take longer than conventional surgery, the pros usually outweigh the cons. Procedures that have recently been improved by the use of robotic technology include hysterectomy (removal of the uterus) and heart valve replacement.

3-SECOND DOSE
Minimally invasive surgery is performed through tiny incisions instead of larger openings, which means patients tend to have quicker recovery times and less discomfort than with conventional surgery.

3-MINUTE TREATMENT
Robotic surgery, also known as computer-assisted surgery, further enhances minimally invasive surgery. Surgeons use robotic arms or computers to manipulate instruments rather than control them manually. The robotic and computer systems feature magnified 3-D high-definition vision and instruments that bend and rotate far more than the human hand. As a result, surgeons can operate with greater vision, precision, and control.

3-SECOND BIOGRAPHY
HANS CHRISTIAN JACOBAEUS
1879–1937
Swedish physician who pioneered laparoscopy and thoracoscopy, and also advocated endoscopic training for medical practitioners

EXPERT
Gabrielle M. Finn

Advances in minimally invasive surgical techniques, and the increased use of robotics, have been hugely beneficial for patients.

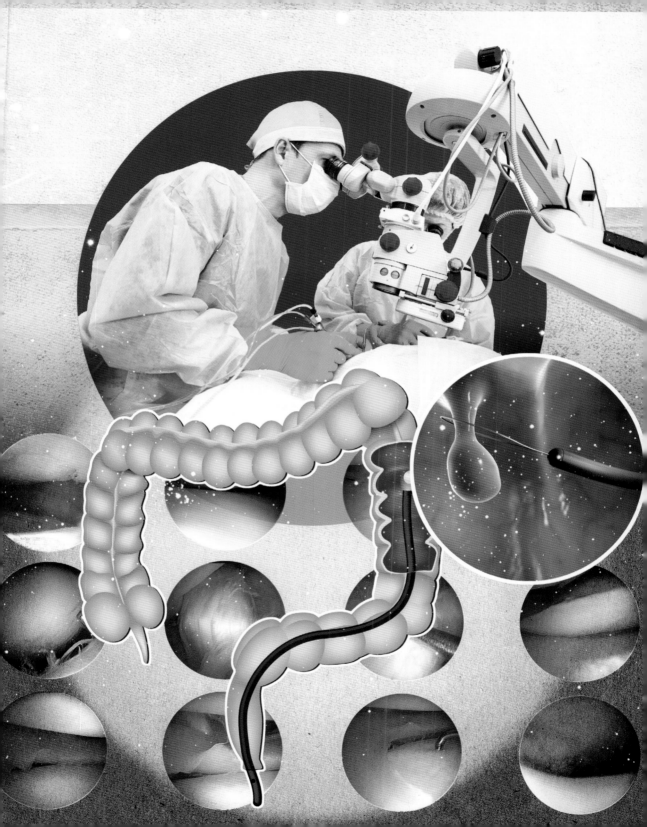

IMAGING & TECHNOLOGY

blastocyst An embryo at around five to six days post-fertilization.

electric field The area near any electrically charged object. It is also known as the electrostatic field.

electromagnetic radiation (EM) A form of energy that is everywhere. It takes many forms, such as radio waves, microwaves, X-rays, and gamma rays. Visible light is also a form of electromagnetic radiation.

flat plate radiograph An imaging technique used when the subject is lying flat. The most common example is an abdominal X-ray.

grafting A procedure that involves taking healthy skin, bone, or other tissue from one part of the body to replace diseased or injured tissue removed from another part of the body. Skin grafts are a common example; grafts are frequently used to treat burns to the skin.

ionizing radiation A radiation that, during an interaction with an atom, can remove tightly bound electrons from the orbit of an atom, causing the atom to become charged or ionized. This type of radiation includes X-rays and gamma rays.

magnetic field A region around a magnetic material or a moving electrical charge within which the force of magnetism acts.

muscle innervation The nerve supply of a muscle. Innervation of a muscle by a nerve brings about the muscle's movement.

myoelectric prosthetics Externally powered artificial limbs that are controlled with the electrical signals generated naturally by the wearer's own muscles.

obstetrics The branch of medicine and surgery concerned with pregnancy, childbirth, and midwifery.

phantom limb A sensation often experienced by amputees that the missing limb is still attached to the body. This sensation is often perceived as pain or that the limb is moving.

piezoelectric crystal A type of crystal that produces a potential difference across its opposite faces when under mechanical stress. Quartz is an example of a piezoelectric crystal.

piezoelectric effect The production of electricity or electrical charge by applying a mechanical stress to certain types of crystals.

radiodensity The inability of electromagnetic radiation, particularly X-rays, to pass through certain materials.

radio wave An electromagnetic wave that has a wavelength between 1/25 inch (1 millimeter) and 18.6 miles (30,000 meters), or a frequency between 10 kilohertz and 300,000 megahertz. It is used for long distance communication.

soft tissue Term that refers to the following tissues of the body: tendons, ligaments, fascia, skin, fibrous tissues, fat, synovial membranes (connective tissue), muscles, nerves, and blood vessels.

sound wave The pattern of disturbance caused by the movement of energy traveling through a medium, such as air, liquid, or any solid matter, as it spreads away from the source of the sound.

tissue regeneration The process of renewal and growth of tissues.

ultraviolet light (UV) A form of radiation that is not visible to the human eye. It is in an invisible part of the electromagnetic spectrum.

X-RAY

In 1895 Wilhelm Röntgen

produced and detected a previously unknown form of electromagnetic radiation now known as X-rays. He observed that when passed through a structure these X-rays were attenuated (reduced in intensity) to varying degrees, based on the density of the object, and could cast shadows on pieces of film. The discovery of X-rays and their penetrating ability was a great revolution in the field of medicine; for the first time the inside of the body could be made visible without invasive surgery. An X-ray image, also referred to as a radiograph, is produced by placing a patient in front of a photographic film or digital detector and exposing the area of interest to a short X-ray pulse. Dense parts of the body, such as bone, stop X-rays from reaching the detector and consequently appear whiter on the image; softer structures, such as the lungs, allow more X-rays to pass through and appear darker. Very soon after their initial discovery X-rays were being used, and still are, for the diagnosis and treatment of patients. They are particularly useful for examining bones and joints, with breaks and fractures being visible, but are also used to detect problems associated with soft tissues such as breast cancer and heart problems.

3-SECOND DOSE
X-rays are a form of electromagnetic radiation that can pass through the body, making them ideal for seeing inside structures.

3-MINUTE TREATMENT
X-rays cannot be seen by the naked eye, or felt, but they have enough energy to disrupt molecular bonds and damage living cells. Due to this ionizing ability, they can be harmful on frequent exposure so special measures are needed to shield patients and medical staff. Their ability to damage cells, however, means they can also be utilized to kill cancer cells, treating cancer using radiotherapy.

RELATED ENTRIES
See also
COMPUTED TOMOGRAPHY (CT)
page 52

RADIOTHERAPIST
page 122

3-SECOND BIOGRAPHIES
WILHELM RÖNTGEN
1845–1923
German physicist who was the first to discover the X-ray; he won the first Nobel Prize in Physics in 1901

JOHN MACINTYRE
1857–1928
Scottish doctor who, in 1896, only one year after the discovery of X-rays, set up the world's first radiology department at the Glasgow Royal Infirmary

EXPERT
Laura Fitton

Röntgen's discovery of X-rays revolutionized medical diagnosis and treatment. As well as their use for imaging, X-rays are also used in some cancer treatments.

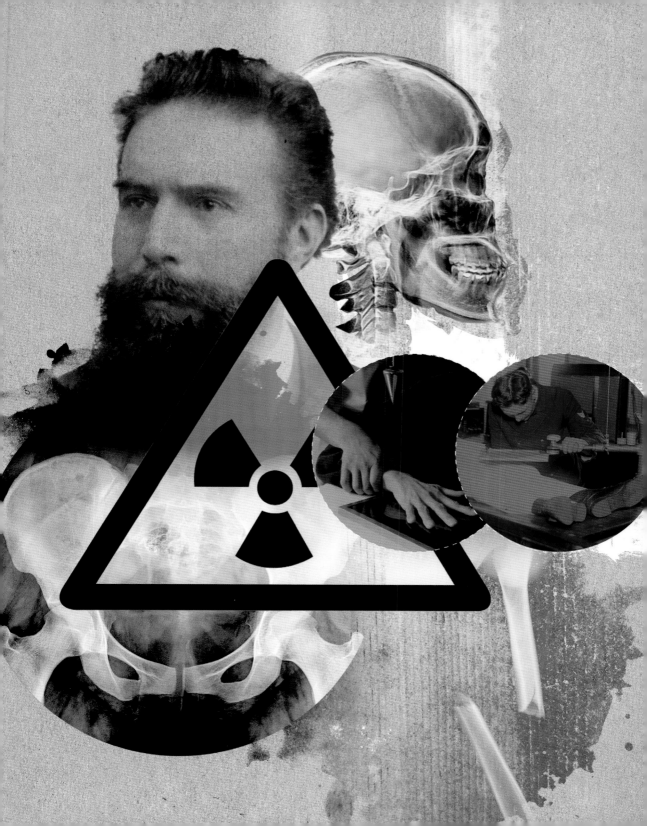

COMPUTED TOMOGRAPHY (CT)

CT scanning was introduced into medical practice in 1971. Computed tomography, which is also referred to as computerized axial tomography (CAT scans), allows for a series of cross-sectional (tomographic) images to be taken, like virtual slices, through a structure or body part. CT scans most commonly use X-rays, but unlike the conventional flat plate radiograph produced with X-rays, 3-D stacks of images are produced. A medical CT scanner uses a rotating X-ray tube and detector. The patient is placed in the scanner and a narrow beam of X-rays is aimed at the patient. Different structures attenuate the X-ray to different extents and 2-D images called tomograms are collected. A computer then processes the series of images allowing the user to see inside the patient without cutting. By setting a threshold value for radiodensity a 3-D model can also be rendered. Compared to traditional radiography (X-rays), CT scans have a high-contrast resolution, allowing tissues that differ in density by small amounts to be distinguished. It also allows for accurate spatial identification of the structure of interest. This means that CT can be used to help diagnose conditions such as broken bones, particularly complex fractures, injuries to internal organs, strokes, and cancer. It can also be used to monitor these conditions and help guide the health professional during a procedure.

3-SECOND DOSE
A CT scan uses a computer and X-rays to create a 3-D image, allowing visualization of internal structures and the diagnosis of many conditions.

3-MINUTE TREATMENT
Patients may often be given a special dye (called a contrast) as a drink, an enema, or injected into the bloodstream to improve the quality and contrast of the CT images. While a CT scan is painless, the ionizing radiation produced by X-rays means there is a moderate to high risk of radiation exposure. This risk, however, will often be minimal compared to the advantages of this diagnostic imaging technique.

RELATED ENTRIES
See also
X-RAY
page 50

3-D PRINTING & BIOPRINTING
page 64

RADIOTHERAPIST
page 122

3-SECOND BIOGRAPHIES
GODFREY HOUNSFIELD
1919–2004
English electrical engineer who invented the first commercially viable CT scanner

ALLAN MACLEOD CORMACK
1924–98
South African physicist; together with Hounsfield, he won the Nobel Prize for Medicine in 1979 for his work on the theory of CT scanning

EXPERT
Laura Fitton

A CT scanner takes a series of cross-sectional "slices" to create a 3-D image. CT scans have a higher contrast resolution than traditional radiographs.

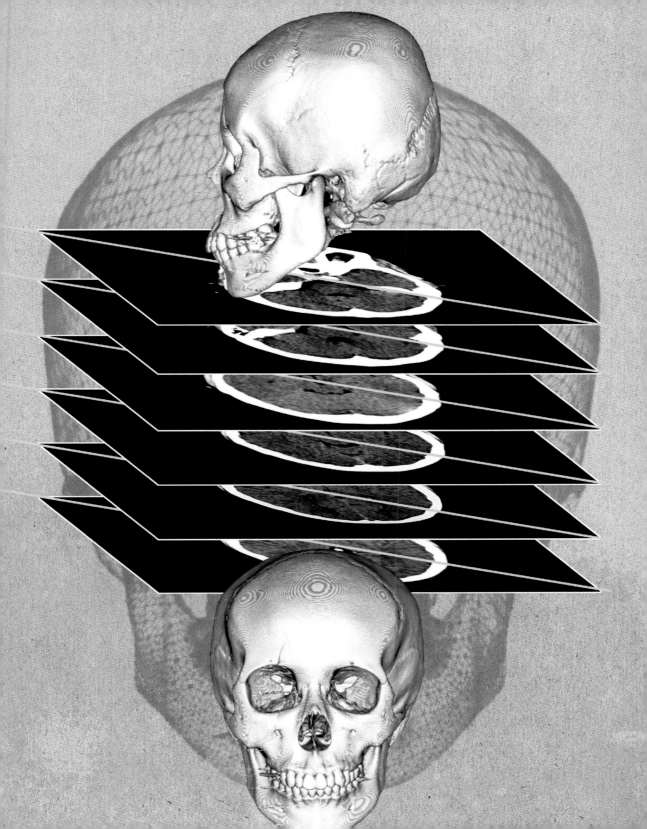

MAGNETIC RESONANCE IMAGING (MRI)

3-SECOND DOSE

During an MRI scan, protons (hydrogen atoms) in tissues containing water molecules are excited to create a signal that is processed to form an internal image of the body.

3-MINUTE TREATMENT

The first human body MRI scan was carried out in 1977, and MRI has since become the most powerful and reliable tool in diagnostic medicine. Unlike CT scanning, MRI does not expose patients to ionizing radiation; therefore, it is often recommended over CT when either approach could yield the same diagnostic information. While safe and painless, it is claustrophobic and not always suitable for people with implants, such as pacemakers, due to the strong magnetic field.

Magnetic Resonance Imaging (MRI) uses strong magnetic fields and radio waves to create internal images of the body. It is particularly useful for medical imaging of soft tissue, including brain and cardiovascular imaging as well as the imaging of internal organs such as the prostate, womb, and liver for diagnostic purposes. Special procedures such as functional MRI (fMRI) also allow brain activity to be measured. An MRI scanner is a large tube surrounded by a superconducting magnet. This magnet can create a magnetic field in the region of 0.5–2.0 tesla, far in excess of the earth's magnetic field. Hydrogen atoms (protons) are very sensitive to changes in magnetic field, and as the human body is mostly made up of water (hydrogen and oxygen atoms), when the patient lies down in the scanner all the body's protons line up in the same direction. Short bursts of radio waves (radiofrequency pulses) are then directed at the region of interest. These pulses excite the atoms, disrupt their alignment, and, when turned off, the protons realign. This sends out signals that are detected by a receiving coil. Protons behave differently depending on the type of material they are found in (for example, fat versus muscle) and realign at different speeds. These signals are then converted into pixels on the computer screen and produce a detailed image of the structure.

RELATED ENTRIES

See also
X-RAY
page 50

COMPUTED TOMOGRAPHY (CT)
page 52

3-SECOND BIOGRAPHIES

NIKOLA TESLA
1856–1943
Serbian-American engineer and physicist who discovered the rotating magnetic field

PETER MANSFIELD
1933–
English physicist credited with introducing mathematical formalism allowing radiofrequency signals to be interpreted as a useful image

EXPERT
Laura Fitton

The most powerful and reliable diagnostic tool available, an MRI uses magnetic fields and radio waves to create images. Specialist MRIs can be used to measure brain activity.

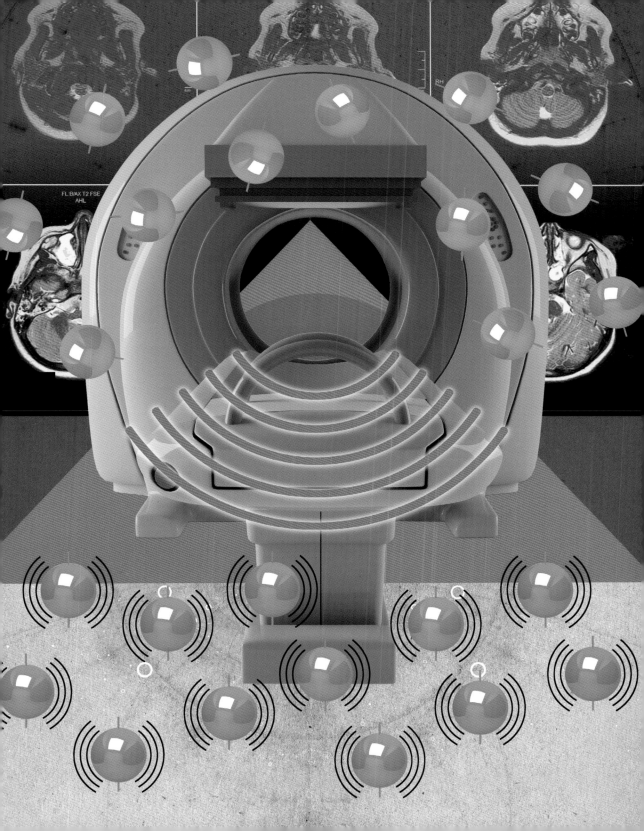

ULTRASOUND

3-SECOND DOSE
Ultrasound produces
real-time images of internal
structures using high-
frequency sound waves.

3-MINUTE TREATMENT
While the potential for
ultrasound in diagnostic
medicine was realized by
the late 1950s, it took until
the 1970s for ultrasound
to be commercially used
in hospitals. It is generally
considered a low-risk
procedure, produces
"live images," and is highly
portable. Limitations,
however, in image quality
are due to the difficulty
sound waves have in
penetrating bone, deep
structures, and passing
through subcutaneous fat
without being attenuated.

Medical ultrasound (also known
as sonography) is a form of imaging modality
that uses ultrasound (sound frequencies greater
than 20,000 hertz, higher than those audible
to humans) to create an image of the inside of
the body. A small probe, called a transducer,
containing piezoelectric crystals, is placed in
contact with the body. When an electric field
is applied the crystals emit high-frequency
sound waves, which are reflected (echoed)
off structures. A real-time moving digital image
is produced with the location and intensity of
each pixel being dependent on how long it takes
the echo to be received after initial transition
and how strong the echo is. Higher frequency
sound waves are not as penetrating and are
therefore used for superficial body structures;
low-frequency sound waves are used for deep
structures. Ultrasound is used as a diagnostic
tool to examine many different body systems,
including internal organs, blood vessels, muscles,
and tendons. A widely used practice is obstetric
ultrasound, producing images of the fetus inside
the mother's uterus. It can also be used to
measure the speed of blood flow. Due to its
heating and disruptive effects, ultrasound also
has therapeutic uses, including the breakdown
of structures such as kidney stones.

RELATED ENTRIES
See also
X-RAY
page 50

COMPUTED TOMOGRAPHY
(CT)
page 52

MAGNETIC RESONANCE
IMAGING (MRI)
page 54

3-SECOND BIOGRAPHIES
PIERRE CURIE
1859–1906
French physicist who
demonstrated the piezoelectric
effect

IAN DONALD
1910–87
Scottish physician who
pioneered the use of diagnostic
ultrasound, in particular to
measure fetal development

EXPERT
Laura Fitton

*Pierre Curie's work on
the piezoelectric effect
led to the development
of ultrasound, which
is particularly useful
for monitoring fetal
development.*

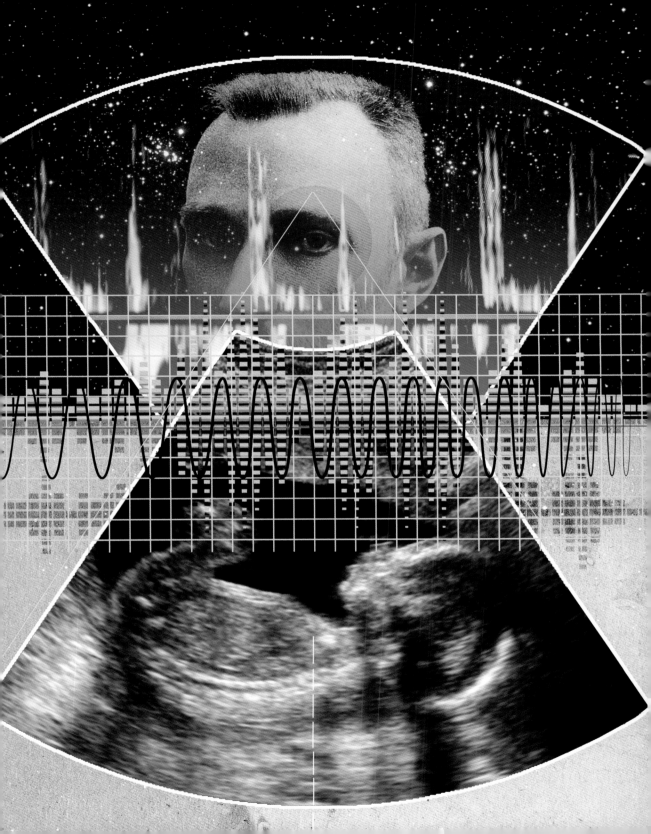

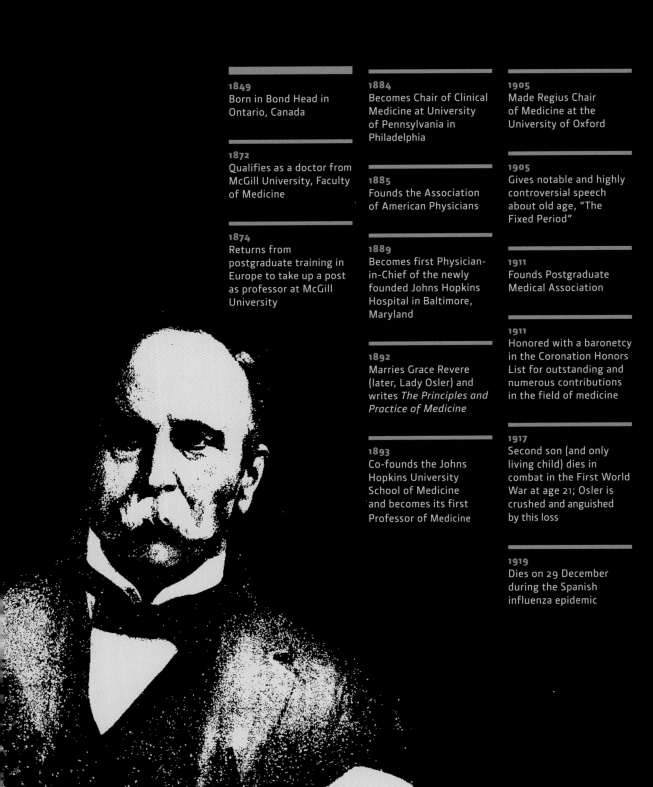

1849
Born in Bond Head in Ontario, Canada

1872
Qualifies as a doctor from McGill University, Faculty of Medicine

1874
Returns from postgraduate training in Europe to take up a post as professor at McGill University

1884
Becomes Chair of Clinical Medicine at University of Pennsylvania in Philadelphia

1885
Founds the Association of American Physicians

1889
Becomes first Physician-in-Chief of the newly founded Johns Hopkins Hospital in Baltimore, Maryland

1892
Marries Grace Revere (later, Lady Osler) and writes *The Principles and Practice of Medicine*

1893
Co-founds the Johns Hopkins University School of Medicine and becomes its first Professor of Medicine

1905
Made Regius Chair of Medicine at the University of Oxford

1905
Gives notable and highly controversial speech about old age, "The Fixed Period"

1911
Founds Postgraduate Medical Association

1911
Honored with a baronetcy in the Coronation Honors List for outstanding and numerous contributions in the field of medicine

1917
Second son (and only living child) dies in combat in the First World War at age 21; Osler is crushed and anguished by this loss

1919
Dies on 29 December during the Spanish influenza epidemic

WILLIAM OSLER

Sir William Osler transformed the way medicine was taught by bringing medical students to the patient's bedside instead of having them learn medicine in lecture theaters. In teaching hospitals, ward rounds led by an experienced physician with a handful of medical students or trainees in tow became the norm as a result of his vision. Medical education was transformed by this new emphasis on the importance of clinical experience in treating patients.

Osler was a man of varied interests: he loved books, had a passion for the history of medicine, and owned a large collection of historical books. He wrote extensively and was a serial practical joker. Early in his career, he identified a component of blood that was previously observed but not fully understood, and demonstrated that this component was a type of blood corpuscle (later named platelets).

Born in Bond Head in Canada to deeply religious parents, Osler initially intended to dedicate his life to the ministry but opted for a medical career instead, starting his medical training at a private institute before transferring to McGill University, from where he qualified in 1872. At the toss of a coin later in his career, Osler accepted the position of Professor of Medicine at a new medical school in the United States—Johns Hopkins University Medical School—and there he joined the chiefs of pathology, surgery, and obstetrics and gynecology to transform the organization and curriculum of clinical teaching.

Osler penned a book *The Principles and Practice of Medicine* (1892), which was a leading textbook in medical circles for an extended period of time. Osler also had a more humorous side and, under the pseudonym Egerton Yorrick Davis, a retired US army surgeon, wrote bizarre hoax patient case histories (sexual), possibly to illustrate the gullibility of medical readers.

In medical circles, Osler has been immortalized in the names of numerous diseases, and signs and symptoms of illness: Osler's nodes are red, tender swellings of the hand and Osler-Rendu-Weber Disease is a hereditary blood disorder with recurrent nose bleeds. He coined the term pneumonia, which, ironically, may have been present on his deathbed in 1919. Several "oslerisms" (quotations by Osler) illustrate his dedication to medical education and patient care. "The good physician treats the disease; the great physician treats the patient who has the disease," is a well-known oslerism. He was created a baronet in 1911 for his numerous contributions to medicine.

Joanna Matthan

STEM CELLS & TISSUE ENGINEERING

3-SECOND DOSE
Stem cells are undifferentiated cells that have the capacity to regenerate and differentiate into specialized cell types.

3-MINUTE TREATMENT
Embryonic stem cells possess enormous therapeutic potential and could lead to new medical treatments including tissue engineering (repairing damaged tissue or even creating new organs); however, controversy surrounds their use. Extraction of embryonic stem cells requires destruction of the blastocyst that subsequently forms the embryo, which means destroying potential life. The ethics of embryonic stem cell research has been questioned, and the production of embryonic stem cell cultures is restricted in some countries.

The human body consists of a vast number of cells that have differentiated into specialized cells (including nerve, skin, blood, bone, and muscle) with varying properties and functions. These cells have lost their ability to generate different forms of cells, but there are also others, known as stem cells, which can self-renew, are less differentiated, and can give rise to various cell types. These properties make stem cells essential for the regeneration needed during our lifetime due to ageing, loss, and damage, but also to construct the body during its initial development from an embryo. Unipotent stem cells, such as skin stem cells, can only produce cells of one type, but they are still regenerative. Embryonic stem cells are pluripotent, meaning they can differentiate into almost any cell type. Stimuli picked up by the stem cells' membrane and nuclei about environmental and genetic factors will trigger a stem cell to differentiate. Scientists are using this to culture stem cells under controlled conditions and steer their differentiation. Tissue regeneration is an important application of stem cell research. Sheets of skin are already being engineered and grafted onto burn victims, stem cells found in blood and bone marrow are used to treat leukemia, and new treatments for Parkinson's and Alzheimer's are looking promising, all through the use of stem cells.

RELATED ENTRY
See also
3-D PRINTING & BIOPRINTING
page 64

3-SECOND BIOGRAPHIES
ERNST HAECKEL
1834–1919
German biologist who was the first to use the term stem cell

JAMES THOMSON
1958–
American developmental biologist who was the first to isolate human embryonic stem cells in 1998

SHINYA YAMANAKA
1962–
Japanese stem cell researcher who discovered that mature cells can be reprogramed to become pluripotent, circumventing an approach in which embryos would be destroyed

EXPERT
Laura Fitton

Stem cells' ability to regenerate and differentiate is already utilized for several treatments and could be applied to other diseases in the future.

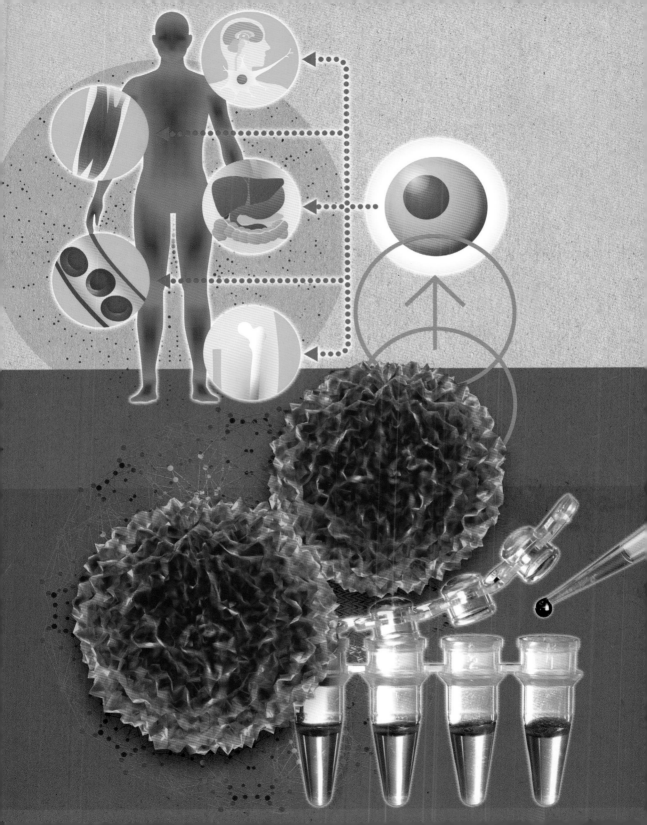

ARTIFICIAL LIMBS

Prosthetics have been used in some form throughout history, from wooden toes in ancient Egypt to iron hands in medieval Europe. While the materials used today, such as plastics and carbon-fiber composites, are more advanced, the basic idea of prosthetics has stayed the same; a prosthetic limb is an artificial device that replaces a missing limb. A team of health care professionals, from psychiatrists to surgeons and prosthetists, are all involved in the rehabilitation of patients following the loss of a limb. Different types of prosthetics are designed with different goals in mind and therefore vary in their suitability. A cosmetic prosthesis (cosmesis) is designed for appearance rather than controllability. Functional prosthetic limbs are designed for usability. The most basic functional limbs are body powered; the desired motion is transmitted to the prosthetic via a system of cables and harnesses attached to a functioning limb, but prosthetics can now be controlled electronically. Recent advancements include myoelectric prosthetics and the inclusion of microprocessors, enabling the imitation of natural behavior, creating bionic limbs that look and move realistically. Mind-controlled prosthetics are also now a thing of reality; using wireless brain implants and targeted muscle re-innervation, patients can even control the movements of their artificial limb through their own thoughts.

3-SECOND DOSE
Cutting-edge prosthetics are now allowing patients to move artificial limbs, in much the way as their original hand or arm, using thought control.

3-MINUTE TREATMENT
Targeted muscle innervation not only allows for fine control of movements of robotic limbs but also provides some sensory feedback. This approach works by splitting a remaining muscle, removing its nerve supply, and rerouting the residual nerves to it. When the patient thinks of moving their phantom limb these re-innervated muscles contract. This activation is picked up by electrodes and used to control the prosthetic.

RELATED ENTRIES
See also
BIONIC ORGANS
page 42

3-D PRINTING & BIOPRINTING
page 64

3-SECOND BIOGRAPHIES
MARCUS SERGIUS
fl. c. 218–201 BCE
Roman general during the Second Punic War and the first documented user of a prosthetic hand; his metal hand was constructed to hold a shield

TODD KUIKEN
1961–
Creator of the bionic arm; he developed the technique of targeted muscle re-innervation, enabling amputees to control motorized prosthetic devices using their minds and to regain sensory feedback

EXPERT
Laura Fitton

Artificial limbs have been used for centuries, but the materials and technology have advanced to allow greater and more natural function.

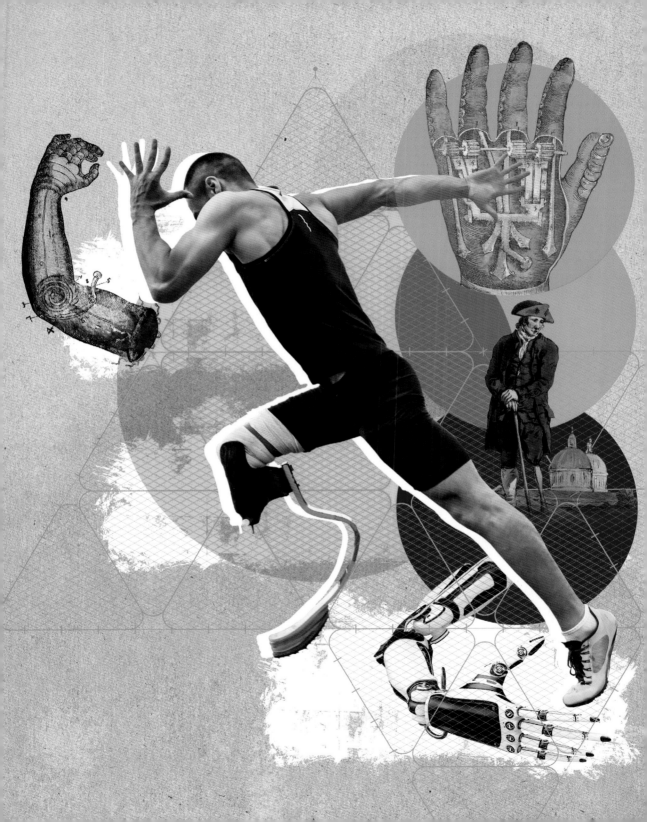

3-D PRINTING & BIOPRINTING

3-SECOND DOSE
3-D printing is a revolutionary technology already being used in medicine today, allowing for custom-made implants and helping to guide surgeries.

3-MINUTE TREATMENT
Incredible uses of 3-D printing in the medical field have already been developed. This includes skin graft printing, the bioprinting of cartilage, blood vessels, bone, heart valves, ear cartilage, custom-made prosthetic parts, and medical equipment. While the full printing of functioning organs has yet to be successfully carried out, medical researchers are well on their way to making this a reality.

A recent major advance in the field of medicine is the use of 3-D printing. Surface scans, produced from various imaging modalities including CT scans, are enabling surgeons to create and print 3-D models of various parts of the body. 3-D printing works by printing ink, which is both substrate and substance, in successive layers to build up a 3-D solid model. 3-D printing was first developed in the 1980s. At this time the ink was acrylic liquid, which turned solid when exposed to ultraviolet light. Now the "ink" comes in a variety of forms including wax, metal, plastics, and living cells. It has already become common for surgeons to use 3-D printed plastic models to practice surgical procedures on. Following CT scanning, the internal architecture of a patient's body can be rendered and used to print custom 3-D models to help design, plan, and trial surgical options. As well as being used externally, 3-D prints are also used to create personalized prosthetics, such as those made from titanium alloys, which can be implanted into the patient. The biggest leap forward for 3-D printing still lies ahead with the printing of full working organs; however, bioprinting has already become a reality. By combining 3-D printing with tissue engineering, bioprinted cells have successfully been dispensed onto biocompatible scaffolds, building living sculptures.

RELATED ENTRIES
See also
COMPUTED TOMOGRAPHY (CT)
page 52

STEM CELLS & TISSUE ENGINEERING
page 60

ARTIFICIAL LIMBS
page 62

3-SECOND BIOGRAPHIES
CHARLES HULL
1939–
Inventor of the first form of 3-D printing, the first rapid prototype technology

STEPHEN POWER
1985–
The first trauma patient to undergo reconstructive surgery using 3-D models and printing

EXPERT
Laura Fitton

3-D printing and bioprinting are new technologies that are already revolutionizing modern medicine, allowing doctors to create custom models.

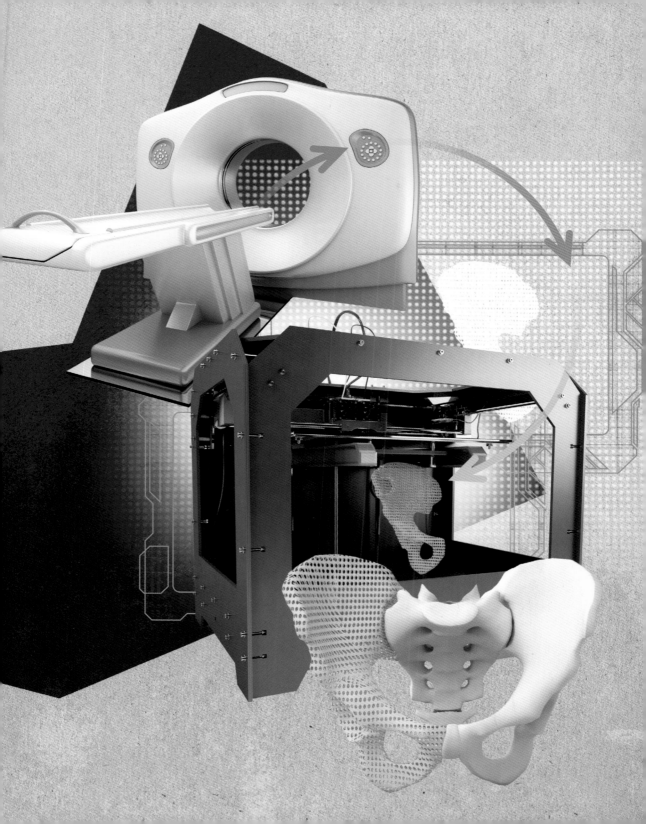

TREATMENTS, THERAPIES & PROCEDURES

TREATMENTS, THERAPIES & PROCEDURES
GLOSSARY

antibody A large Y-shaped protein. Antibodies are recruited by the immune system to identify and neutralize foreign substances such as bacteria and viruses. Each antibody has a unique target known as the antigen present on the invading organism (for example, bacteria or virus).

antigen A toxin or other foreign substance that induces an immune response in the body, especially the production of antibodies.

aseptic An environment or procedure that is free from contamination caused by harmful bacteria, viruses, or other microorganisms. Surgically sterile environments aim to be aseptic to prevent infection in a patient.

bacteria The simplest of creatures that are considered alive. They are microscopic living organisms, usually one-celled, that can be found everywhere. They can be dangerous, and cause infection, or beneficial in processes such as digestion.

barber-surgeons Medical practitioners in medieval Europe who, unlike many doctors of the time, performed surgery, often on the war-wounded. A barber-surgeon would normally learn his trade as an apprentice to a more experienced colleague. Many would have no formal learning, and they were often illiterate.

immune system A system of the body that protects against disease. The immune system must detect a wide variety of agents, such as viruses and bacteria, that could cause harm to the body and fight them off.

leukocyte *See* white blood cells.

palliative surgery A form of surgery used to improve a patient's quality of life by easing pain or other symptoms caused by advanced or untreatable cancer. It is not used as a cure or treatment for cancer.

pathogen An infectious, biological agent that is a cause of disease or illness to its host.

pessary A small soluble block of a drug that is inserted into the vagina either to treat infection or as a contraceptive. Alternatively, a vaginal pessary can be a removable plastic device placed into the vagina to help to support areas of pelvic organ prolapse.

plasma The liquid part of the blood and lymphatic fluid, which makes up about half of the volume of blood. Plasma is devoid of cells. Blood plasma contains antibodies and other proteins. It is taken from donors and made into medications for a variety of blood-related conditions.

platelets Tiny pieces of blood cells that help wounds heal and prevent bleeding by forming blood clots. Platelets are made in bone marrow.

psychosurgery The neurosurgical (brain surgery) treatment of mental disorder. Psychosurgery has always been a controversial medical field.

psychotropic medication The term for any medication capable of affecting the mind, emotions, and behavior of a patient.

red blood cells Also called erythrocytes, red blood cells are the most common type of blood cell. They are the body's principal means of delivering oxygen to its tissues. Red blood cells also remove carbon dioxide from the body, transporting it to the lungs to be exhaled. Red blood cells are made in the bone marrow. They typically live for about 120 days, and then they die.

virus A biological agent that reproduces inside the cells of living hosts. Infected host cells are forced to produce many thousands of identical copies of the original virus, at an extraordinary rate. This replication of the virus can cause the host to become ill, such as a human with the cold or flu virus.

white blood cells Also called leukocytes, white blood cells are the cells of the immune system that are involved in protecting the body against both infectious disease and foreign invaders.

IMMUNIZATION & VACCINATION

RELATED ENTRY

See also
POLIO
page 102

Immunization is a natural process of resistance to pathogens (bugs causing illness) that has been harnessed for use to prevent the deadly effects of infectious diseases. It can occur naturally when a person is exposed to an infectious agent, such as chicken pox, or can happen artificially with a vaccine. Immunity to a pathogen is brought about by targeting antibody proteins that recognize a specific part of the pathogen (the antigen) and make it ineffective (neutralization). Immunity to a pathogen can happen either actively or passively. In active immunization the effects are long-lasting because the person's own immune system is stimulated to produce antibodies: after recovering from an episode of mumps, for example, the person is immune to re-infection by the mumps virus because their immune system recognizes the virus and produces antibodies that neutralize it. This can also be induced by vaccination. Vaccines contain weakened or killed forms of pathogens that can stimulate the same response but do not cause illness. Passive immunization involves giving antibodies produced by another person's immune system; the effects are immediate but short-lived. Most countries have vaccination programs to ensure the most vulnerable in society (children and immunocompromised people) are safe from harmful infections.

3-SECOND BIOGRAPHIES

EDWARD JENNER
1749–1823
English physician, pioneer of smallpox vaccination, and father of immunology who inserted cowpox pus into a cut on an eight-year-old boy's (James Phipps) arm and proved he was immune to smallpox

LOUIS PASTEUR
1822–95
French chemist and microbiologist who in 1881 demonstrated that immunization against anthrax was possible by injecting sheep with a modified form of *Bacillus anthracis*; he also developed a protective concoction against the deadly rabies virus

EXPERT
Joanna Matthan

The work of pioneers such as Edward Jenner led to the development of successful vaccination programs.

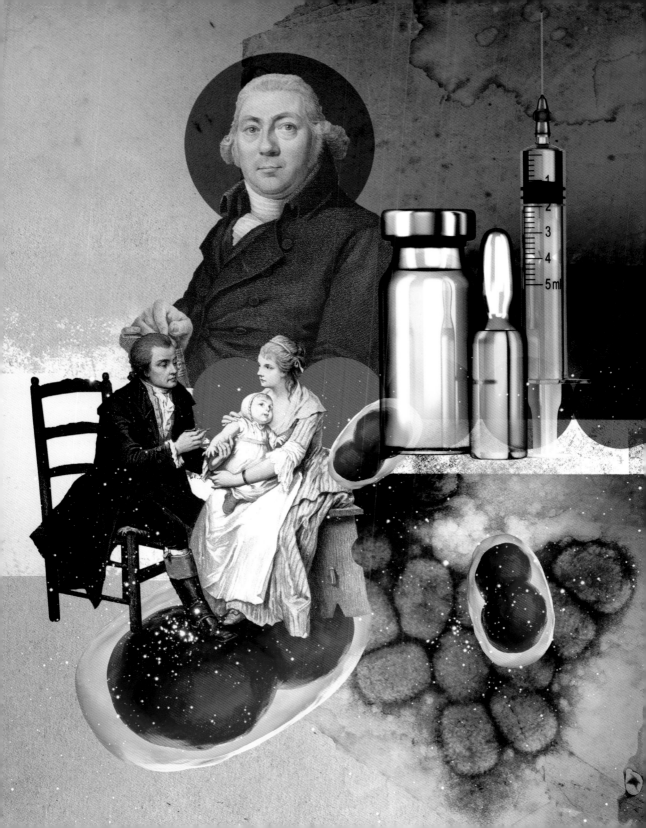

CANCER TREATMENTS

3-SECOND DOSE
Cancer treatment is usually tailored to an individual and can include surgery, radiotherapy, chemotherapy, or a combination of treatments to be effective.

3-MINUTE TREATMENT
Early cancer treatments were sometimes too terrible to think about. Barber-surgeons conducted operations in unhygienic conditions without pain relief, leaving patients disfigured or dead, and useless concoctions were offered to those suffering from debilitating illness. Improvements in sanitation and surgical techniques (asepsis), treatment of wound infections (antibiotics), diagnostic imaging (X-ray, MRI, CT), and availability of pain relief (anesthetic agents) mean cancer sufferers now have improved chances of surviving and being cured.

After a diagnosis of cancer, a treatment plan will be quickly developed by a multidisciplinary specialist team. The conventional treatment options are surgery, radiotherapy, chemotherapy, or a combination of any of those and, depending on the type of cancer, its spread, speed of spread, and condition of the patient, the specific treatment will be selected. Surgery is a good option when the disease has not spread beyond the site it originated from, and can be curative. It can also be used to lessen pain (palliative surgery) or improve function (if a tumor is blocking the intestine, for example). Radiotherapy destroys cancer cells and about half of cancer patients will receive radiotherapy (surgery is more common and the two are often combined to ensure the margins around tumors have been tackled). Cancer cells are far more sensitive to radiation than healthy cells, and the radiation causes them to commit cell suicide (apoptosis) or to be genetically damaged so they cannot replicate. Chemotherapy chemically destroys cancer cells. Unwanted effects arise from all these treatments; however, as chemotherapeutic agents kill healthy cells in addition to cancer cells, the effects are more widespread (nausea, hair loss, anemia). Chemotherapy can also result in a life-threatening loss of the white cells that fight infection (neutropenic sepsis).

RELATED ENTRIES
See also
COMPUTED TOMOGRAPHY (CT)
page 52

MAGNETIC RESONANCE IMAGING (MRI)
page 54

ANESTHESIA & SURGERY
page 80

CANCER
page 106

3-SECOND BIOGRAPHIES
WILLIAM STEWART HALSTED
1852–1922
American surgeon who developed the radical mastectomy for breast cancer

EMIL GRUBBE
1875–1960
American homeopathic physician who used radiation to treat breast cancer

EXPERT
Joanna Matthan

A treatment plan for cancer can incorporate a range of treatments and therapies to target tumors.

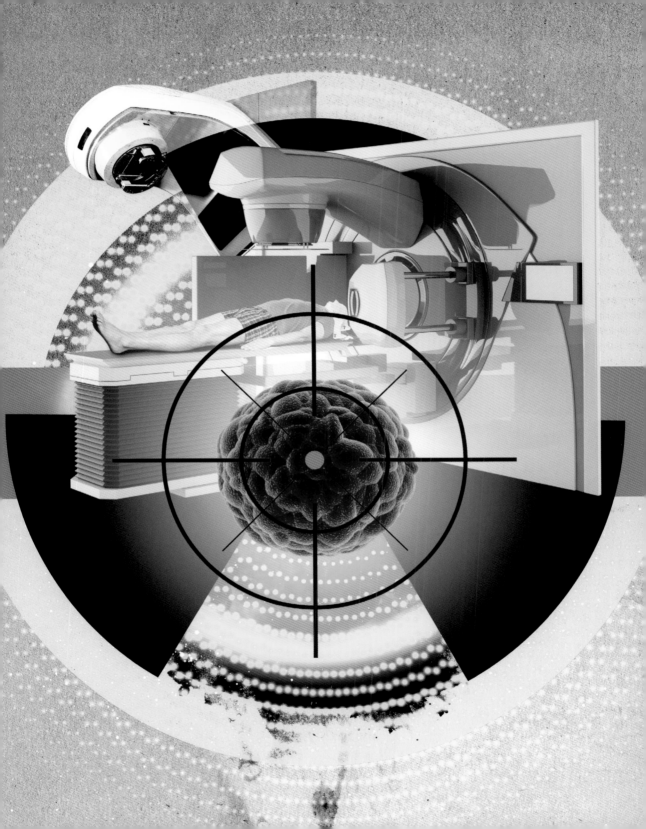

CONTRACEPTION

3-SECOND DOSE
Contraception is any
one of a number of
methods or devices used
to prevent pregnancy.

3-MINUTE TREATMENT
Contraception was
documented, and fairly
successful, in ancient Egypt
(pessaries of crocodile
dung, obscure herbs, and
honey were recommended),
but it was only in the late
nineteenth century that a
greater variety of more
reliable contraceptive
methods started being
used widely. One of the
oldest, and not hugely
reliable, methods
of contraception is
withdrawing the penis
before sperm is ejaculated
(coitus interruptus).
It is widely used in
cultures or religions
where contraception
is not permitted.

Contraception or birth control

is deliberate avoidance of pregnancy, and is achievable today by a variety of methods. The most reliable methods for preventing pregnancy are those that are fairly permanent and virtually irreversible, in other words, sterilization: cutting off the connection between the tube that transmits sperm from the testicle to the penis (vasectomy) in males and clamping the uterine tubes (tubal ligation) in women are 99 percent reliable. Reversible and 99 percent reliable methods of contraception are hormonal contraceptives (birth control pills), intrauterine devices (plastic or metal objects that cause mild inflammation and thus prevent the phases of fertilization), and condoms that are used with a spermicide, if they are used in the correct manner. Many have a small risk of unwanted effects, such as weight gain, nausea, blood clots, and pelvic inflammatory disease. Truly safe, side-effect free methods include avoiding sex during the period around ovulation and using barrier devices (condoms, spermicides, diaphragm, and cervical cap) and breast-feeding regularly after delivery—these are not reliable methods, however. Contraception has played a major role in controlling populations, and the condom has also helped to control the spread of sexually transmitted infections.

RELATED ENTRY
See also
HUMAN IMMUNODEFICIENCY
VIRUS (HIV)
page 104

3-SECOND BIOGRAPHIES
SORANUS OF EPHESUS
fl. 1st/2nd century CE
Greek physician who wrote *On Midwifery and the Diseases of Women*, the most detailed early account of contraception

ALETTA HENRIETTE JACOBS
1854–1929
Dutch physician and inventor who was committed to providing women with contraception and wrote the first systematic work on contraception

JOHN ROCK
1890–1984
American obstetrician and gynecologist who played a major role in developing the first hormonal birth control pill; he also pioneered sperm freezing and IVF

EXPERT
Joanna Matthan

Contraceptive methods and devices vary in reliability but all aim to prevent pregnancy.

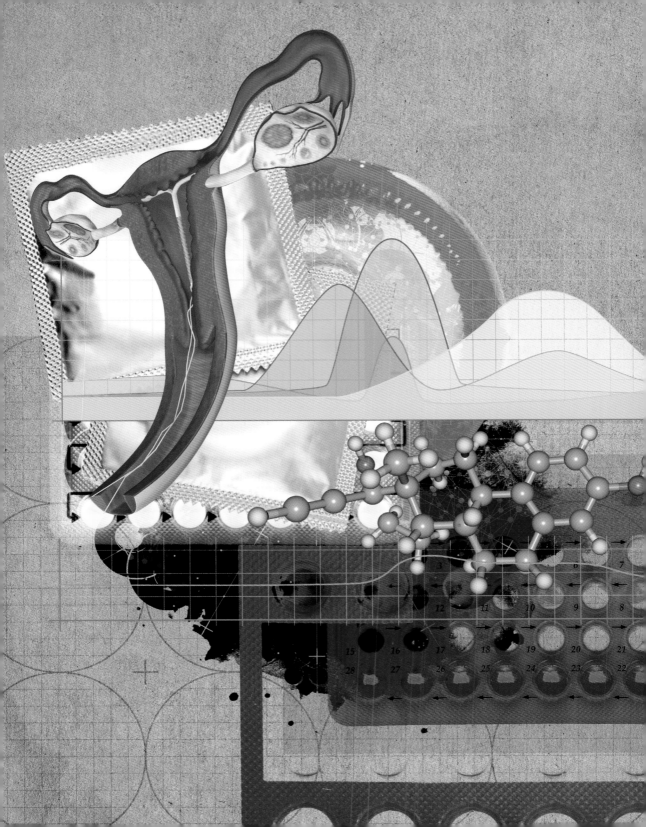

ANTIBIOTICS

RELATED ENTRIES
See also
JOSEPH LISTER
page 38

ALEXANDER FLEMING
page 78

ANESTHESIA & SURGERY
page 80

3-SECOND DOSE

Antibiotics have revolutionized medical pharmacology and are widely used today to treat and prevent infections resulting from numerous types of bacteria.

3-MINUTE TREATMENT

Ancient Egyptians, Greeks, and Indians, among others, used specific molds to treat infection. It was only after Alexander Fleming isolated the mold called *Penicillium* that the truly positive and revolutionary effects of antibiotics began to be appreciated. An excellent example is the treatment of the sexually transmitted disease syphilis. Prior to antibiotics, contracting syphilis was a death sentence, with patients descending into madness in the late stages. One dose of penicillin cures the illness.

Antibiotics are chemically made drugs (derived from mold) that can kill or stop the growth of bacteria. They are widely used to treat infections caused by bacteria, such as inflamed appendices, tuberculosis, wound infections, syphilis, and so on. Sometimes they are used to prevent bacterial infections, especially in those who have undergone a surgical procedure (to prevent wound infection) or in those with a weakened immune system. Antibiotics are completely ineffective against viruses, so organisms that cause influenza and the common cold cannot and should not be treated with them. Antibiotics are designed to take advantage of the difference between the structure of the host's cell and the bacterial cell. They can prevent multiplication of bacterial cells so that the population stays low and the host is able to defend itself better (macrolides and tetracyclines), or they can kill bacteria by preventing them from building their cell walls (penicillins and sulphonamides). Narrow-spectrum antibiotics (Penicillin G) target specific bacteria, and broad-spectrum antibiotics (tetracyclines) are effective against a wide range of organisms. Widespread use of antibiotics has caused much concern in the medical community, as more and more bacteria have become resistant to antibiotics, and infections are becoming increasingly difficult to treat.

3-SECOND BIOGRAPHIES
JOHN SCOTT BURDON-SANDERSON
1828–1905
English physician and physiologist who observed that *Penicillium* (mold) stopped the growth of bacteria

ALEXANDER FLEMING
1881–1955
Scottish biologist, pharmacologist, botanist, and Nobel Prize winner who was the first to grow a pure culture of mold of the *Penicillium notatum* species in 1928, later concentrated into what he termed penicillin

EXPERT
Joanna Matthan

Derived from molds, antibiotics are used to treat infections caused by bacteria.

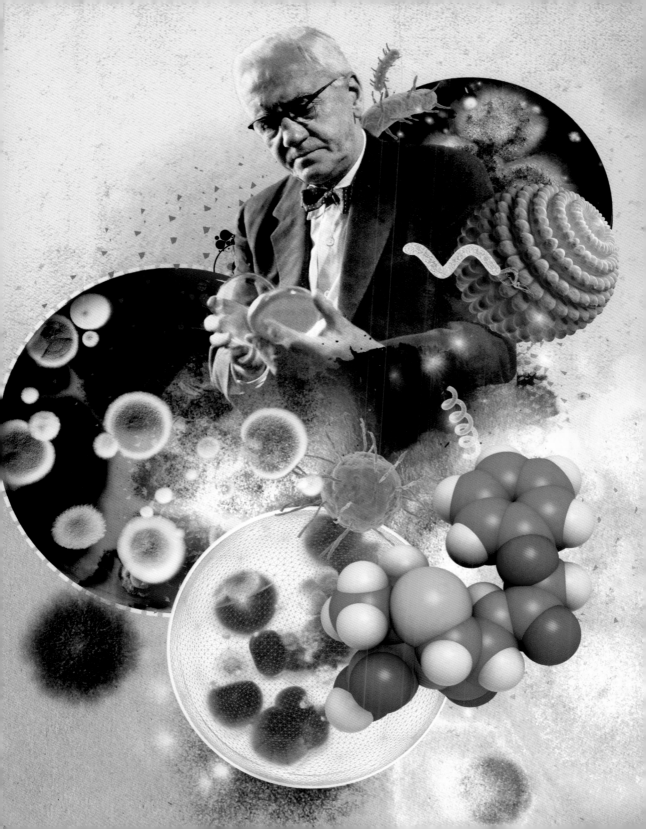

1881
Born in Lochfield, Scotland

1903
Enrols in St Mary's Hospital Medical School, London

1906
Qualifies as a doctor, with distinction, and begins training for a surgical career

1908
Gains BSc degree with Gold Medal in Bacteriology and becomes lecturer at St. Mary's (until 1914)

1909
Becomes a fully fledged surgeon but continues to look for ways to treat infection

1914–18
Serves in the First World War as Captain in the Royal Army Medical Corps; notes how wound infection worsened using antiseptic agents

1921
Discovers lysozyme, an enzyme in bodily fluids with a natural antibacterial effect

1928
Discovers penicillin (*Penicillium notatum*); elected Professor of Bacteriology

1929
Publishes first report on penicillin in the *British Journal of Experimental Pathology*; continues experimenting with penicillin and gives it up in 1940 (Howard Florey and Ernst Boris Chain take up researching it at Oxford Radcliffe Infirmary and later mass-produce it after the bombing of Pearl Harbor)

1943
Elected Fellow of Royal Society (FRS)

1945
Receives Nobel Prize in Physiology or Medicine (shared with Florey and Chain)

1948
Elected Emeritus Professor of Bacteriology, University of London

1951
Elected Rector of University of Edinburgh (a three-year term)

1955
Dies of a heart attack and now rests in St. Paul's Cathedral in London

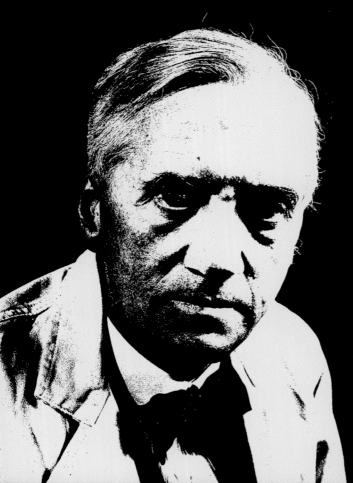

ALEXANDER FLEMING

Alexander Fleming's quiet discovery in 1928 of the mold *Penicillium notatum*, which had accidentally contaminated a culture dish of *Staphylococcus* bacteria he had been growing in his messy laboratory (and caused the bacteria to stop growing), places him amongst the most influential people of the twentieth century. He published his findings in 1929 but received little enthusiasm from the medical world initially, and spent the next 11 years desperately trying to isolate and cultivate the mold. When he finally gave up the struggle in 1940, two scientists at Oxford University, Howard Florey and Ernst Chain, continued to research penicillin and developed it so it could be used as a drug. It was mass-produced in the 1940s to help the war-wounded. Fleming later named the antibiotic penicillin, after calling it "mold juice" for want of a better word. His discovery of an antibiotic agent that could stop killer bacterial illnesses from progressing has saved countless lives worldwide and changed the course of history.

Fleming was born in Ayrshire in 1881 and was the son of a Scottish farmer. When he was 16, he moved to London to work in the shipping industry. After inheriting some money, he decided to train as a doctor. Fleming was an exceptional student, and qualified with distinction from St. Mary's Hospital Medical School in 1906. He stayed on at the school and began a research career in bacteriology under Sir Almroth Wright (a pioneer in immunology and vaccine therapy), and obtained a BS in Bacteriology and was awarded a Gold Medal.

Fleming served in the First World War as Captain in the Royal Army Medical Corps and continued to make significant observations on the treatment of deep wound infections. During this turbulent period, in 1915, he married a trained Irish nurse, Sarah McElroy, and had one son, Robert, with her. He returned to St. Mary's after the war. After his wife's death in 1949, he remarried a Greek colleague at St. Mary's, Amalia Koutsouri-Vourekas, in 1953.

Throughout his extremely productive life, Fleming wrote countless papers on immunology, bacteriology, and chemotherapy and received numerous awards. He was knighted by King George VI in 1944, just after being elected Fellow of the Royal Society in 1943. The culmination of a lifetime of achievements came in 1945 when he shared the Nobel Prize in Medicine with Florey and Chain. He died of a heart attack on March 11, 1955.

Joanna Matthan

ANESTHESIA & SURGERY

Anesthetic agents are used to numb sensation or induce sleep during certain tests or surgical procedures and, in this way, these medications reduce pain and discomfort for the patient. Local anesthetics numb a small area and are used for minor procedures. The patient is awake for the process. A general anesthetic induces total unconsciousness and is used for major operations. Anesthesia can also be used to numb larger areas while keeping the patient awake (such as epidural anesthesia during labor and delivery). Without effective anesthesia, modern-day surgery would be impossible. Each branch of surgery has numerous sub-specialties. Surgeons do elective surgery for non-life-threatening conditions. Emergency surgery is done immediately to save life or limb, and semi-elective surgery is needed to avoid permanent damage but can be postponed. Surgeons sometimes opt to do explorative surgery to help confirm a diagnosis. Today, surgical procedures are done in teams made up of surgeons, their assistants (a junior doctor), anesthetists, scrub nurses, and theater assistants. Procedures vary in length depending on the nature and difficulty of the procedure—mole removal can be done in minutes, for example, while the removal of a part of the intestine can take hours. Patients need to be anesthetized and aseptic conditions ensured.

3-SECOND DOSE

Most surgical procedures would not be possible without effective anesthesia (numbing agents) and experienced anesthetists overseeing the well-being of patients.

3-MINUTE TREATMENT

Surgery has been performed for centuries and was highly developed in some civilizations, such as ancient India and China. In Europe, surgeons began to be trained in universities in the 1700s and became part of the medical profession. Their anatomical knowledge allowed them to do procedures quickly (amputations could be done within minutes) but without anesthetic agents, the specialty did not grow. This changed with increased understanding of germ theory and asepsis, and the availability of imaging (X-ray) and anesthetic agents.

RELATED ENTRIES
See also
ORIGINS OF MEDICINE
page 16

JOSEPH LISTER
page 38

X-RAY
page 50

CANCER TREATMENTS
page 72

3-SECOND BIOGRAPHIES
HUMPHRY DAVY
1778–1829
British chemist and inventor who in 1798 demonstrated that inhalation of nitrous oxide (laughing gas) relieved pain

WILLIAM THOMAS GREEN MORTON
1819–68
American dental surgeon who demonstrated publicly in 1846 that surgical anesthesia could be successful by using ether during an operation

EXPERT
Joanna Matthan

The development of effective anesthestics made modern-day surgery possible.

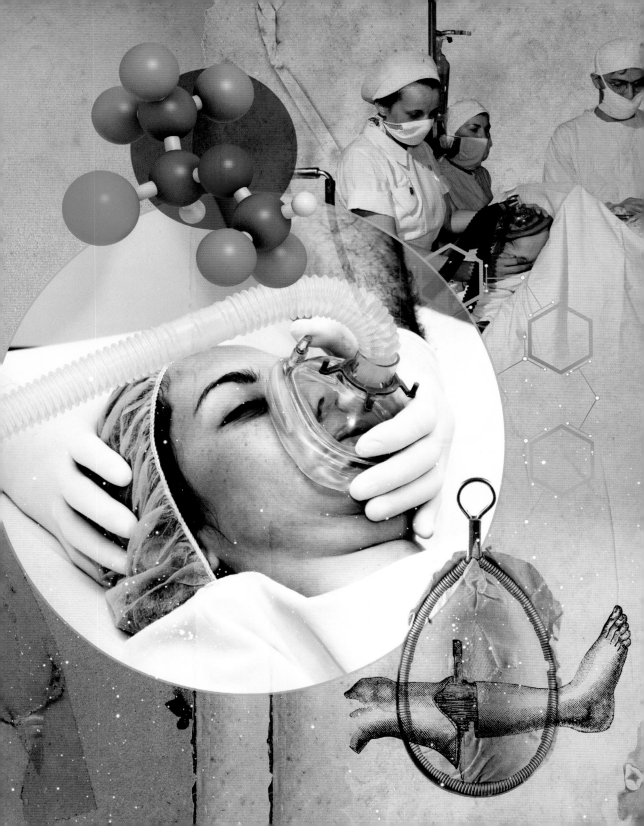

BLOOD TRANSFUSION & DONATION

3-SECOND DOSE
Medicine depends on
blood donations from
unpaid volunteers who
donate their blood so
that blood transfusions
can take place during
emergency or routine
medical procedures.

3-MINUTE TREATMENT
In the mid-seventeenth
century, Europeans tried
out blood transfusions but
countless patients died
from incompatibility
reactions. Today, blood
transfusions are frequent
and lifesaving procedures
but were not safe until
the ABO and Rh (Rhesus)
blood group systems were
identified. In the 1970s,
blood transfusions were
found to pose a significant
risk of transmitting
life-threatening viruses
(hepatitis B/C, HIV). Since
then, donor blood has been
tested for antibodies to
the most common viruses.

The transfer of blood from one
person (donor) into the vein of another person
(recipient) is known as a blood transfusion.
Modern medicine relies on blood transfusions
for countless routine and emergency procedures,
and a constant source of donations is required
as the lifespan of blood products is very short.
There are over 35 recognized blood group
systems, but the two most important ones are
the ABO and the RhD antigen systems. A person
can be one of four blood types (A, B, AB, O)
and additionally either Rh (rhesus) positive or
negative; classification is based on the presence
or absence of an antigen (a protein or
carbohydrate) on the surface of the red blood
cell. Both parents contribute to a person's blood
type. Donor blood (from unpaid volunteers in
most countries) is screened to ensure the blood
they are donating is safe. The blood is separated
into different components (red blood cells,
plasma, white blood cells, and platelets) and
each component is used based on recipient
need. Blood is transfused over a long period of
time (a unit of red blood cells takes four hours
to transfuse and platelets take 30 minutes).
This is to ensure the safety of the recipient. It is
not uncommon to have undesirable reactions to
transfusion, which may happen for many reasons
such as allergy, sensitivity to donor leukocytes,
or undetected red-cell incompatibility.

RELATED ENTRIES
See also
ORGAN DONATION
& TRANSPLANT
page 30

STEM CELLS & TISSUE
ENGINEERING
page 60

3-SECOND BIOGRAPHIES
KARL LANDSTEINER
1868–1943
Austrian-American physician
and biologist who discovered
the main blood groups and
developed the modern
classification of blood groups

JAN JANSKY
1873–1921
Czech neurologist, psychiatrist,
and serologist who first
classified blood into the
ABO blood group system

EXPERT
Joanna Matthan

*Blood transfusions
are essential for many
medical procedures —
the four blood types
are determined by the
antigens present or
absent on the red
blood cell.*

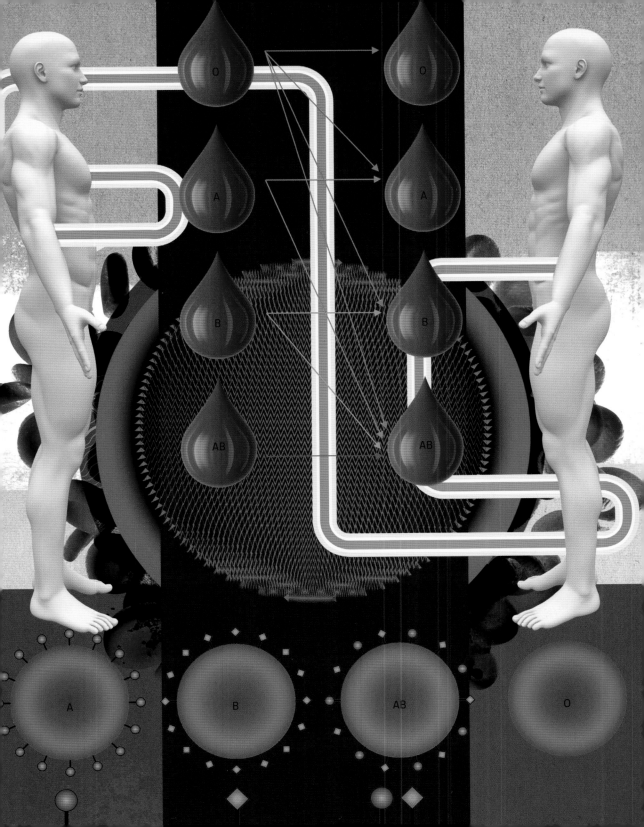

LOBOTOMY & ELECTROCONVULSIVE THERAPY (ECT)

RELATED ENTRIES
See also
ANESTHESIA & SURGERY
page 80

PSYCHOTHERAPY
page 86

3-SECOND DOSE
Lobotomy and ECT were widely used for incurable mental illness in a time when medication to control psychiatric illness was not available.

3-MINUTE TREATMENT
Widespread public awareness of the negative effects of ECT and lobotomies was raised as a result of Ken Kesey's novel *One Flew Over the Cuckoo's Nest* (1962). The main character (faking insanity) is lobotomized and left in a vegetative state. The book and subsequent film adaptation in 1975 captured the public imagination and both procedures were heavily criticized and fell into decline. Even at the peak of their popularity, many psychiatrists and psychotherapists opposed the use of lobotomies and ECT.

Cutting the connection between the frontal lobes and the rest of the brain, known as lobotomy, was first performed in the 1930s. As patients with mental disorders were thought to have fixed circuits within the brain, it was believed that cutting the connection could change their behavior. Two holes were drilled on the top or the sides of the skull and a leucotome (a sharp instrument) was pushed into the brain and swept from one side to the other between the frontal lobes (the front part of the brain) and the rest of the brain. This psychosurgical procedure made its way into mainstream psychiatry and was used to treat compulsive disorders, depression, mania, and schizophrenia. Thousands of operations were performed every year, but it fell out of favor in the 1950s because of its poor and debilitating results for the patients who received it. Electroconvulsive therapy (ECT, shock treatment) is still used to treat intractable mental illness such as severe depression. It was introduced by two Italian doctors in 1938. The procedure involves passing alternating electrical current from either side of the temples via electrodes. This leads to immediate unconsciousness and a seizure. It is followed by some memory loss, and is given as a course over a few weeks. Since the discovery of tranquilizing drugs, its use has decreased.

3-SECOND BIOGRAPHIES
GOTTLIEB BURCKHARDT
1836–1907
Swiss physician and psychiatrist who performed the first psychosurgical operation

EGAS MONIZ
1874–1955
Portuguese neurologist, co-founder of modern psychosurgery, inventor of lobotomy

WALTER JACKSON FREEMAN II
1895–1972
Performed the first lobotomy in the US; his "ice-pick" method allowed quick access through the back of the eye-sockets into the brain

EXPERT
Joanna Matthan

Now superseded by medications, lobotomy and ECT used to be the main treatments for mental illnesses.

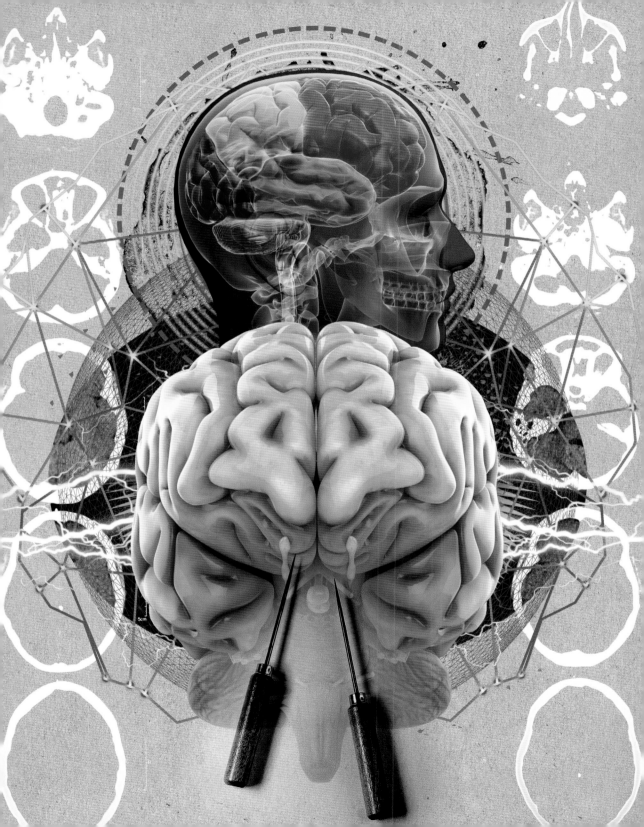

PSYCHOTHERAPY

Psychotherapy is an umbrella

term used for a host of counseling methods aimed at treating emotional, psychological, and behavioral disorders. A trained therapist establishes a safe and intimate relationship with the person (or group) requiring therapy, aiming to identify, change, and remove the disturbing symptoms and promote personal well-being. Psychotropic medications may be used, but the patient's response to the therapist's words is where true change occurs. Psychotherapeutic methods include exploring problems, emotional support, and behavior therapies, which aim to treat challenging behaviors and emotional states by using countermeasures based on Ivan Pavlov and B. F. Skinner's theories on conditioning as well as Albert Bandura's social learning theory. Psychological suffering was previously thought to be caused by evil spirits and was treated by priests and medicine men. In the 1800s, Franz Anton Mesmer demonstrated that troublesome psychiatric symptoms disappeared when a patient was under a trance, and so began the attempt to scientifically understand the human mind. Sigmund Freud and Josef Breuer observed the link between traumatic childhood experiences and developing mental illness at a later date. Freudian psychoanalysis incorporated a method of "talking cure," which has hugely influenced modern psychotherapy.

3-SECOND DOSE

Psychotherapy (counseling) is any one of a wide set of talking therapies used to treat those with emotional, psychological, or behavioral disorders.

3-MINUTE TREATMENT

The work of the early psychoanalysts has influenced psychotherapy and psychology, and also filtered into literature and art. Sigmund Freud popularized the terms unconscious, conscious, and conscience through his theory of psychological reality (id, ego, and superego). Words from his writings have slipped into our everyday vocabulary when we use terms such as neurotic, denial, libido, cathartic, anal, repression, and Freudian slips; our ideas on sexuality and personality disorders have stemmed from his life work.

RELATED ENTRY

See also
SHAMANS & WITCH DOCTORS
page 14

3-SECOND BIOGRAPHIES

IVAN PAVLOV
1849–1936
Russian physiologist and Nobel Prize winner most well-known for his classical conditioning work and the concept of conditioned reflex which he demonstrated in salivating dogs

SIGMUND FREUD
1856–1939
Austrian neurologist and founder of psychoanalysis; possibly the greatest contributor to exploring the secrets of the human mind

ALBERT BANDURA
1925–
American psychologist who penned social learning theory, the basis for modern psychotherapy

EXPERT

Joanna Matthan

Modern psychotherapy is still influenced by the research and theories of Freud and Pavlov.

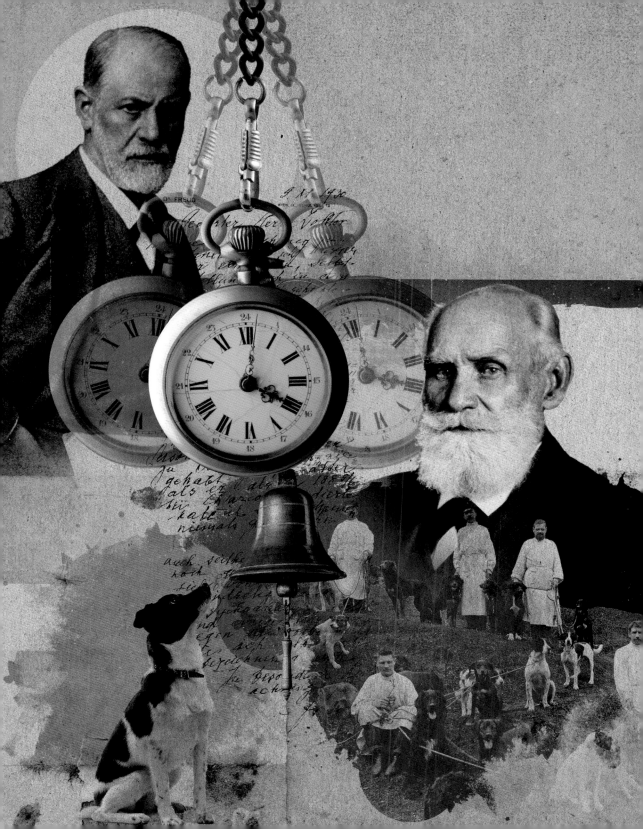

DISEASES

DISEASES
GLOSSARY

aneurysm An excessive localized swelling of the wall of an artery. An aneurysm is caused by a weakness in the blood vessel wall, usually where it branches.

antibiotics Medications used to treat or prevent bacterial infections.

artery A tube (blood vessel) that carries blood high in oxygen content away from the heart to the rest of the body.

blood sugar The concentration of glucose in the blood. Glucose is a sugar that comes from the foods we eat, and it's also formed and stored inside the body. It's the main source of energy for the cells of our body, and is carried to each cell through the bloodstream.

central nervous system The central nervous system (CNS) is the part of the nervous system consisting of the brain and spinal cord.

endemic disease Refers to the constant presence of diseases or infectious agents within a particular geographical area or population group.

gene therapy An experimental technique that uses genes to treat or prevent disease. There are three main mechanisms:
1 Replacing a mutated (permanently altered) gene that causes disease with a healthy copy of the gene,
2 Inactivating, or "knocking out," a mutated gene that is malfunctioning, and
3 Introducing a new gene into the body to help fight a disease.

immune system A system of the body that protects against disease. The immune system must detect a wide variety of agents, such as viruses and bacteria, that could cause harm to the body and fight them off.

lymph vessel Another name for lymphatic vessels, which are thin-walled, valved structures that carry lymph around the body.

physiotherapy A medical discipline that helps restore movement and function when someone is affected by injury, illness, or disability. Physiotherapists help people through movement and exercise, manual therapy, education, and advice.

protozoan Protozoa are defined as single-celled organisms with animal-like behaviors, such as motility and predation.

stroke A serious, life-threatening medical condition that occurs when the blood supply to part of the brain is cut off. They can occur if a blood clot blocks a vessel in the brain or if a vessel bursts.

virus A biological agent that reproduces inside the cells of living hosts. Infected host cells are forced to produce many thousands of identical copies of the original virus, at an extraordinary rate. This replication of the virus can cause the host to become ill, such as a human with the cold or flu virus.

MALARIA

Among the diseases affecting

humans, malaria has had one of the largest impacts. Estimated by some researchers to have killed up to half of all humans who have ever lived, malaria remains one of the greatest dangers to health today, with around 200 million cases and an estimated 600,000 deaths each year. Malaria is caused by five species of the protozoan *Plasmodium*, which undergo part of their life cycle in mosquitoes of the genus *Anopheles*. Infection occurs when an infected mosquito bites a person to take a blood meal. The symptoms of malaria usually start one to three weeks after infection and include fever, headache, vomiting, and jaundice. In severe cases, malaria can lead to seizures, coma, or death. Even after apparently successful treatment of malaria, patients may suffer a recurrence of symptoms several months later. Historically, malaria was treated with quinine, a drug derived from the bark of the cinchona tree, but nowadays the standard treatment is artemisinins, drugs isolated from the sweet wormwood plant and combined with other antimalarials. Despite much research, no vaccine currently exists, and malaria remains endemic in over one hundred countries in tropical and subtropical regions of the world.

3-SECOND DOSE

Malaria is an infectious disease caused by a parasitic protozoan and transmitted by mosquitoes, causing over half a million deaths each year.

3-MINUTE TREATMENT

Owing to the high levels of mortality it causes, malaria has been suggested to be one of the greatest selective pressures on human evolution in modern times. A number of genetically inherited diseases persist at high rates in the population in malarial areas because being a carrier for these conditions provides a degree of resistance against malaria. These include blood disorders such as sickle cell disease and thalassemia.

3-SECOND BIOGRAPHIES

CHARLES LOUIS
ALPHONSE LAVERAN
1845–1922
French physician who discovered that malaria was caused by a parasitic protozoan, the first time protozoans had been shown to be the cause of any disease

RONALD ROSS
1857–1932
British physician who proved that malaria was transmitted by mosquitoes; he received the Nobel prize for Physiology or Medicine in 1902

TU YOUYOU
1930–
Chinese medical scientist who extracted artemisinin, used to treat malaria, from the sweet wormwood plant; she received the Nobel prize for Physiology or Medicine in 2015

EXPERT
Philip Cox

Malaria is a highly infectious disease that is spread by mosquitoes. It is widespread in tropical and subtropical areas.

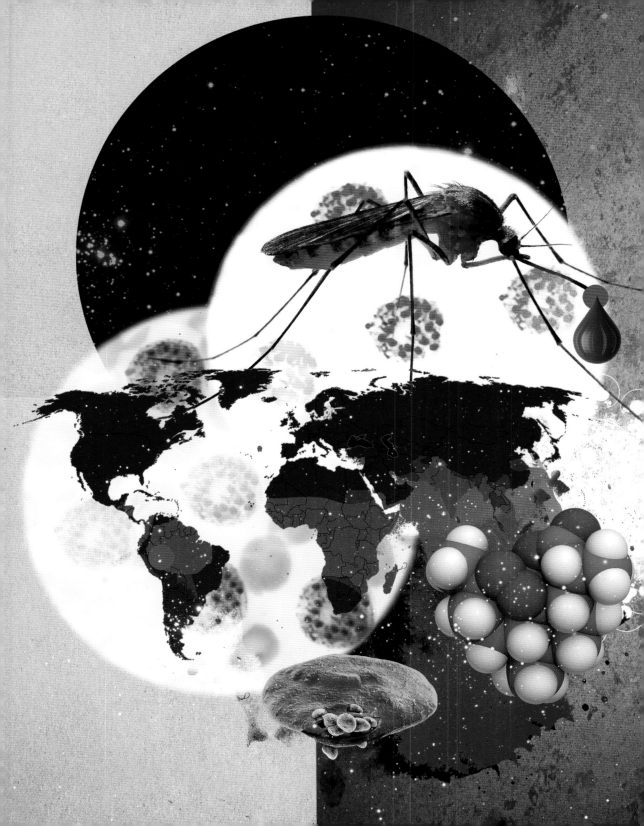

DEMENTIA

Dementia affects parts of the brain responsible for language, memory, and decision-making. It can cause devastating changes to the personality of those who suffer with it. Most cases of dementia are caused by disease and cannot be reversed. There have been links made between dementia and alcohol and drug abuse. There are a number of different diseases that cause dementia; Alzheimer's is the most common. Patients with Alzheimer's have a build-up of protein in the brain; these are known as plaques. Plaques result in a loss of connections between nerve cells in the brain—eventually leading to the death of brain tissue. Other types include vascular dementia and dementia with Lewy bodies. Vascular dementia is caused by reduced blood supply to the brain due to diseased blood vessels. There are many types of vascular dementia—stroke is a common cause. Dementia with Lewy bodies is caused by deposits of abnormal proteins called Lewy bodies inside brain cells in areas of the brain responsible for things such as memory and muscle movement. Typically, dementia cannot be cured and tends to get worse over time. Eventually, dementia patients need help with all day-to-day activities and can require 24-hour care. There are some medications that can be given to try and delay the progression of the disease and help patients remain independent for as long as possible.

3-SECOND DOSE
Dementia describes symptoms that may include memory loss and difficulties with mental agility, thinking speed, problem-solving, understanding, and language.

3-MINUTE TREATMENT
Alcohol abuse can result in dementia or other syndromes, such as Korsakoff's syndrome. Patients with Korsakoff's syndrome present with dementia-like symptoms such as the loss of short-term memory. Alcohol-related dementia is caused by neurological damage that impairs brain function.

3-SECOND BIOGRAPHY
ALOYSIUS "ALOIS" ALZHEIMER
1864–1915
Bavarian-German psychiatrist and neuropathologist; he first described severe memory loss in a patient, Auguste Deter, which later became known as Alzheimer's disease

EXPERT
Gabrielle M. Finn

Alzheimer's and other forms of dementia affect the parts of the brain that govern language, memory, and decision-making, leading to a gradual and long-term decline in the patient's functioning.

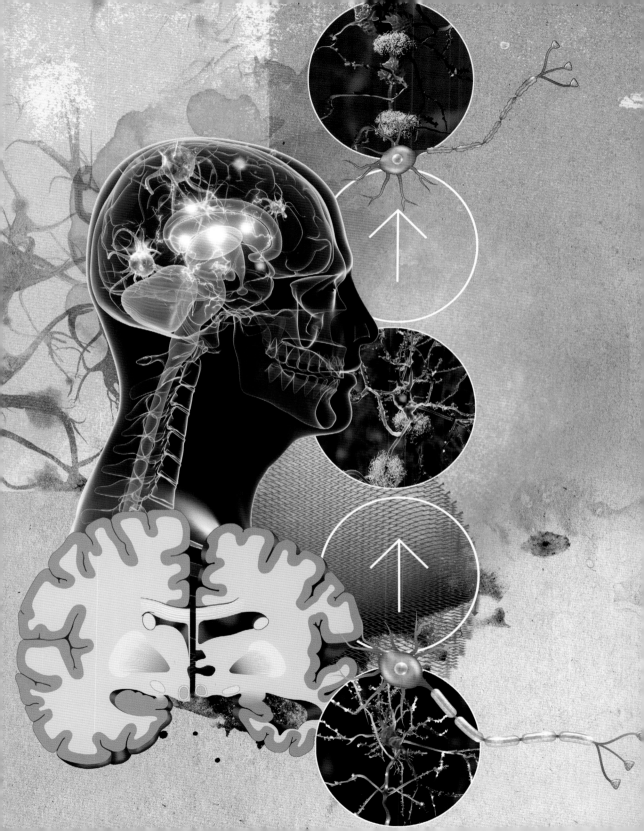

DIABETES MELLITUS

3-SECOND DOSE

Diabetes mellitus, commonly known as diabetes, is a disease in which blood sugar (glucose) levels are high for prolonged periods of time.

3-MINUTE TREATMENT

Some women develop diabetes during pregnancy—this is known as gestational diabetes. Women with gestational diabetes don't have diabetes before their pregnancy and the condition usually goes away after giving birth.

Blood sugar is controlled by

insulin, a hormone secreted by the pancreas. Digested food enters the blood stream as glucose, insulin moves glucose out of the blood and into cells, where it is broken down to produce energy. Diabetics are unable to break down glucose due to a lack of insulin or cells not responding to insulin. Patients with diabetes suffer with high blood sugar (hyperglycemia), which can cause serious damage to organs. Common symptoms of diabetes include thirst, frequent urination, confusion, and weight loss. If a diabetic has too much insulin or not enough sugar, their blood sugar can fall dangerously low; this is known as hypoglycemia. If sugar levels fall too low it can result in a coma. There are different types of diabetes. Type 1, early or child onset, is autoimmune, meaning that the immune system attacks and destroys the cells that produce insulin. Type 1 diabetics are insulin dependent. Type 2 diabetes, late onset, is the most common form and often caused by poor lifestyle, including obesity. In Type 2, insulin is either not produced or cells don't react to it (insulin resistance). Type 2 does not always require insulin—some cases can be controlled by diet and exercise alone. Most diabetics manage their condition by testing their glucose levels and either administering insulin if they are high, or eating sugar if they are low.

RELATED ENTRY
See also
INSULIN
page 140

3-SECOND BIOGRAPHiES
FREDERICK BANTING
& CHARLES H. BEST
1891–1941 & 1899–1978
Canadian doctor (Banting) and his medical student (Best) who discovered insulin; they injected it into a dog and found that it lowered blood sugar levels; Banting was awarded a Nobel Prize for his work, but controversially, Best was not

EXPERT
Gabrielle M. Finn

Banting and Best's discovery of insulin revolutionized the treatment of diabetes. Produced in the pancreas, insulin regulates the body's glucose levels.

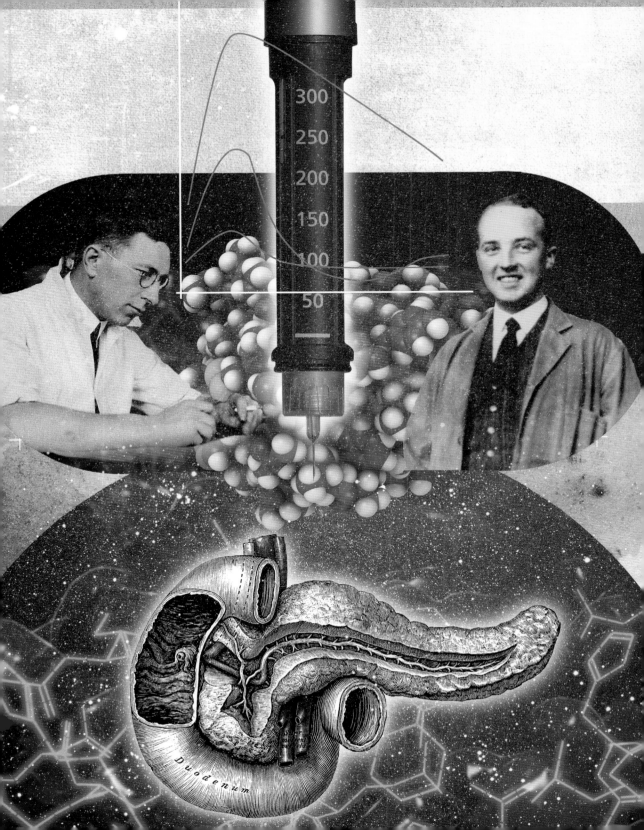

Duodenum

VASCULAR DISEASE

Vascular disease can affect the entire body. Types of vascular disease include Coronary Heart Disease (CHD)—often referred to as Coronary Artery Disease (CAD), Peripheral Artery Disease, stroke, aortic aneurysm, carotid artery disease, pulmonary embolism (blood clots), deep vein thrombosis (DVT), and varicose veins. CHD occurs when the flow of oxygenated blood to the heart is either blocked or reduced by a build-up of fatty deposits (atheroma) in the coronary arteries that supply blood to the heart. Reduced blood flow causes chest pain, known as angina. If the coronary arteries become totally blocked a heart attack, known as a myocardial infarction (MI) can result. Similarly, a stroke occurs when blood flow to the brain is restricted. The sooner a patient receives treatment the better. Drugs can be given to minimize the damage to cells caused by the lack of oxygenated blood. Risk factors for vascular disease include high cholesterol, high blood pressure, a lack of physical activity, diseases such as diabetes, a family history, smoking, and obesity. Treatments depend on the type of vascular disease. Positive lifestyle changes can be effective; some patients may require surgery to open up blocked vessels and others may be prescribed a variety of drugs to alleviate symptoms. Strokes, heart attacks, blood clots, and aneurysms can cause death if extremely severe or not treated quickly enough.

3-SECOND DOSE

Vascular disease includes any condition that affects the circulatory system, caused by inflammation, weakness, or the build-up of fatty deposits in vessels.

3-MINUTE TREATMENT

Aneurysms occur when the wall of an artery weakens allowing it to distend. Aortic aneurysms occur in the large artery (aorta) directly leaving the heart. Cerebral aneurysms occur in the arteries supplying the brain. Both can be fatal.

RELATED ENTRIES

See also
BYPASS & PACEMAKERS
page 34

HUMAN GENOME PROJECT
(HGP)
page 36

BLOOD TRANSFUSION
& DONATION
page 82

ANTICOAGULANTS
page 148

3-SECOND BIOGRAPHY
ANCEL BENJAMIN KEYS
1904–2004
American scientist who discovered links between diet and health, in particular that a high fat diet can cause heart disease

EXPERT
Gabrielle M. Finn

Vascular disease is caused by blood vessels that are inflamed, weak, or clogged with excess fatty deposits.

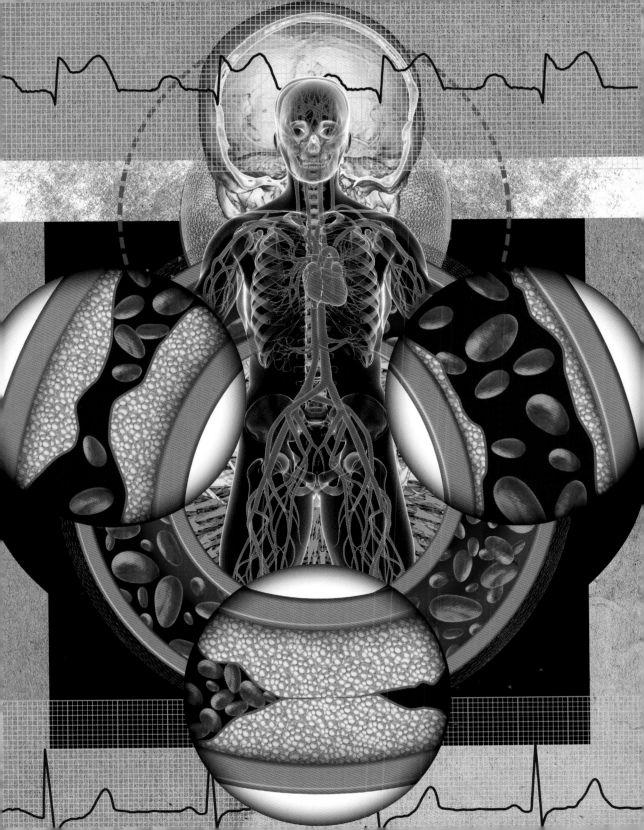

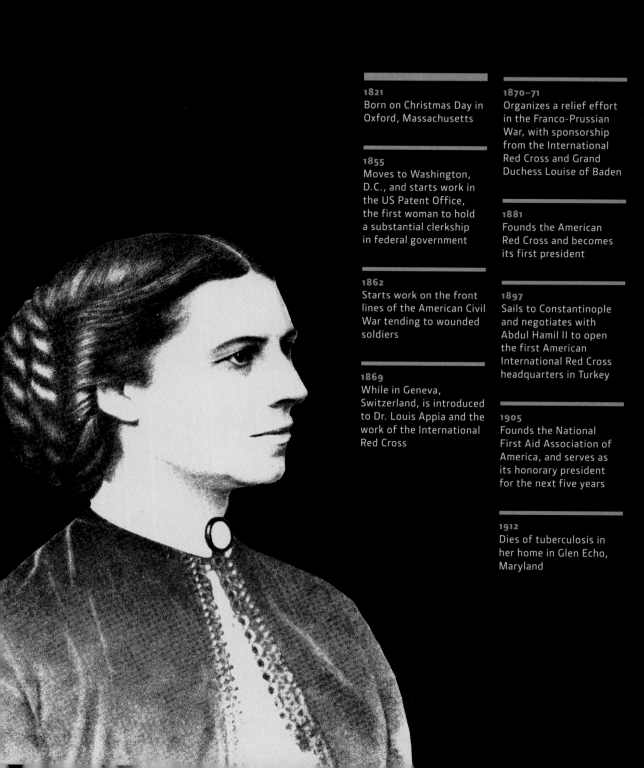

1821
Born on Christmas Day in Oxford, Massachusetts

1855
Moves to Washington, D.C., and starts work in the US Patent Office, the first woman to hold a substantial clerkship in federal government

1862
Starts work on the front lines of the American Civil War tending to wounded soldiers

1869
While in Geneva, Switzerland, is introduced to Dr. Louis Appia and the work of the International Red Cross

1870–71
Organizes a relief effort in the Franco-Prussian War, with sponsorship from the International Red Cross and Grand Duchess Louise of Baden

1881
Founds the American Red Cross and becomes its first president

1897
Sails to Constantinople and negotiates with Abdul Hamil II to open the first American International Red Cross headquarters in Turkey

1905
Founds the National First Aid Association of America, and serves as its honorary president for the next five years

1912
Dies of tuberculosis in her home in Glen Echo, Maryland

CLARA BARTON

Clara Barton was an American nurse and humanitarian who devoted her life to providing aid to people in distress, eventually founding the American Red Cross. Her achievements are all the more notable given her gender and the time in which she lived.

Born in Massachusetts in 1821, Barton spent her early career as a teacher, working in schools in Georgia and Canada, before opening her own free school in New Jersey. However, frustrated that the school board insisted on hiring a man to head the school, Barton left teaching in 1855 and began work as a clerk in the US Patent Office. She was the first woman to do so, although she was dismissed two years later after a change of government. She returned to the office in 1861 and was thus in Washington, D.C., as the American Civil War began.

Initially, Barton provided help to injured soldiers in Washington by gathering much-needed food, clothing, and medical supplies. In 1862, she was finally granted permission to travel to the front lines to attend to the wounded. Her unceasing work in these dangerous conditions over the next three years earned her the name "Angel of the Battlefield."

In 1868, Barton set off on a trip to Europe on the advice of her doctor. While in Switzerland, she was introduced to Dr. Louis Appia and the work of the International Red Cross. With sponsorship from the Red Cross and Grand Duchess Louise of Baden she organized a relief effort to help the wounded soldiers of the Franco-Prussian War. On her return to the USA, Barton began to gather support for the founding of the American Red Cross. By arguing that such an organization was needed to help people affected by natural disasters, not just wars, she was able to convince President Chester Arthur, and the American Red Cross was established in 1881. Although now 60 years old, Barton was elected its president, a role she fulfilled for over 20 years.

In 1904, owing to criticism of her financial management and her age, Barton was forced to resign as president of the American Red Cross. She immediately set her sights on a new project and founded the National First Aid Association of America the following year. She spent her final years in her home in Maryland, where she died of tuberculosis in 1912 at the age of 90.

Philip Cox

POLIO

RELATED ENTRY
See also
IMMUNIZATION
& VACCINATION
page 70

In 1952, the USA experienced its worst-ever polio epidemic. Although the highly infectious viral disease of poliomyelitis is thought to have been present in human populations for thousands of years, its incidence dramatically increased from the beginning of the twentieth century onwards. Most polio infections pass with few or no symptoms, but in a small minority the poliovirus will enter the central nervous system leading to muscle weakness and paralysis, which can be fatal if the respiratory muscles are affected. In the 1952 epidemic, over 3,000 patients died and over 21,000 were left with some degree of paralysis. The American public recognized the urgent need for a vaccine against polio and donated millions of dollars to medical research to find one. Finally in 1955, to great public acclaim, Jonas Salk announced the development of a successful inactivated virus polio vaccine. Its use, alongside the live oral polio vaccine developed by Albert Sabin a few years later, has led to the near extinction of polio. The World Health Organization made polio the subject of a global eradication program in 1988, and at the time of writing the disease remains endemic in only two countries.

3-SECOND DOSE
Polio is an infectious viral disease that, in the severest cases, can lead to paralysis and death. Effective vaccines have almost eradicated it globally.

3-MINUTE TREATMENT
Polio epidemics in the 1940s and 1950s had profound effects on medicine and society. The need for expensive mechanical ventilators ("iron lungs") for patients with respiratory paralysis, led to the foundation of specialist respiratory centers, which were the forerunners of modern intensive care units. Furthermore, the large number of polio survivors with some form of paralysis promoted significant advances in the social and civil rights of disabled people.

3-SECOND BIOGRAPHIES
BASIL O'CONNOR
1892–1972
Head of the National Foundation for Infantile Paralysis who provided backing to Jonas Salk during development of a polio vaccine

ALBERT SABIN
1906–93
Polish-American medical researcher who developed a live attenuated oral polio vaccine; also developed vaccines against encephalitis and dengue fever

JONAS SALK
1914–95
American virologist who developed the first vaccine for polio; founded the Salk Institute for Biological Studies in 1960

EXPERT
Philip Cox

The poliovirus can enter the central nervous system, causing muscle weakness and paralysis.

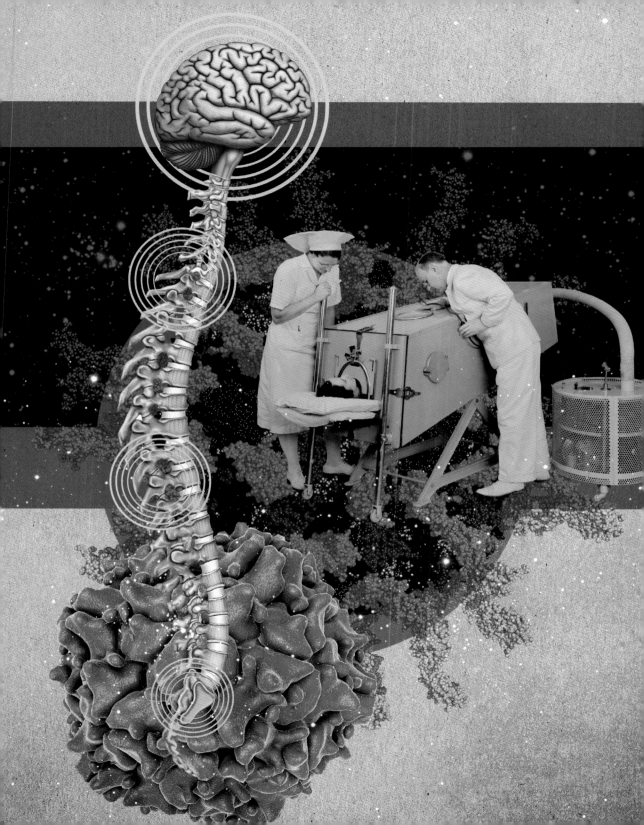

HUMAN IMMUNODEFICIENCY VIRUS (HIV)

HIV is contracted through

contact with the blood or certain body fluids of an infected individual. The virus invades the body's immune system, causing significant damage over time. Eventually the body is unable to fight off infections. HIV enters CD4 cells in the immune system. CD4 cells are responsible for protecting the body against viruses, bacteria, and germs. Once inside the CD4 cells, HIV replicates itself hundreds of times. These copies then leave the CD4 cells, killing them in the process. This sequence continues until eventually the number of CD4 cells drops to such low levels that the immune system stops working; this can take around ten years and a patient may feel perfectly well until this point. The later stages of HIV are referred to as Acquired Immune Deficiency Syndrome (AIDS), characterized by severe infections, weight loss, and skin lesions. Without treatment, around half of HIV patients will develop AIDS within ten years. As yet there is no cure for HIV, but treatments are available to help patients live longer and prevent it from developing into AIDS. Post-exposure prophylaxis (PEP) can be given to people within 72 hours of exposure to the virus to help stop them contracting it.

RELATED ENTRIES
See also
HUMAN GENOME PROJECT (HGP)
page 36

CONTRACEPTION
page 74

BLOOD TRANSFUSION & DONATION
page 82

3-SECOND BIOGRAPHY
LUC ANTOINE MONTAGNIER
1932–
French virologist who discovered the Human Immunodeficiency Virus; he was awarded the 2008 Nobel prize for Physiology or Medicine

EXPERT
Gabrielle M. Finn

3-SECOND DOSE
Human Immunodeficiency Virus (HIV) attacks the body's immune system, weakening its ability to fight infections and disease.

3-MINUTE TREATMENT
HIV is typically passed on through blood and body fluids, including breast milk, semen, vaginal and rectal fluids/linings. HIV is most commonly caught by having unprotected sex. Other common ways of acquiring HIV include sharing infected needles or from a HIV-positive mother during pregnancy, childbirth, or breast-feeding. Urine, sweat, and saliva do not contain enough of the virus to pass it on.

The HIV virus replicates within CD4 cells, damaging the body's immune system and leaving the patient vulnerable to further disease and infection.

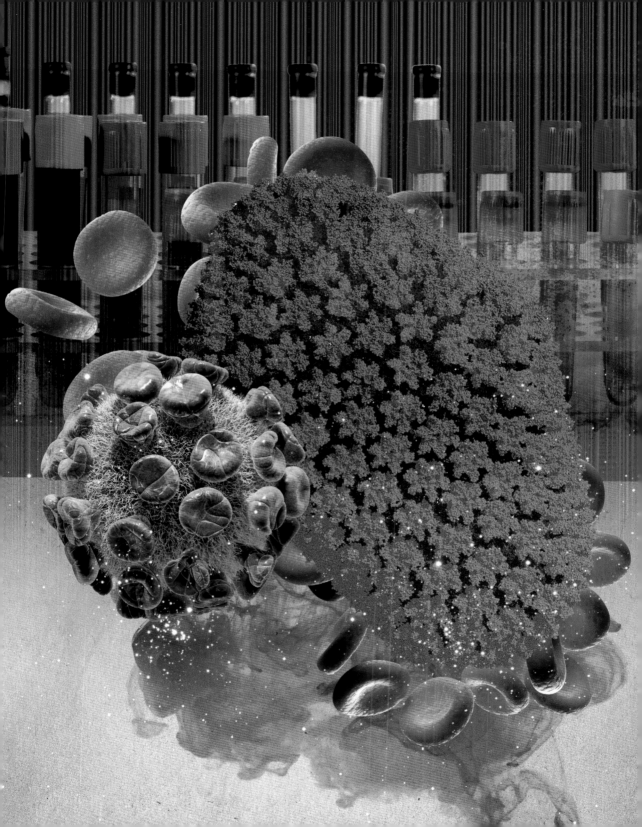

CANCER

There are hundreds of different

types of cancer. Some are inherited, whereas others start when a gene mutates over a person's lifetime. In both cases, abnormal cells replicate and invade the tissues of the body. Cancers are divided into groups according to the type of cell they originate from and include carcinomas, lymphomas, sarcomas, brain tumors, and leukemias. Carcinomas are the most common type—they begin in epithelial cells, which are found in the skin or within tissues that line or cover internal organs. Cancers that start in blood or bone marrow are called leukemias. In addition to unexplained mutations or genetic factors, cancers can also be caused by external factors, such as exposure to certain toxic agents like tobacco or ultraviolet (UV) light. These are known as carcinogens. Carcinogens do not cause cancer all the time but repeated exposure can be detrimental and increase the likelihood of developing cancer. Some cancers can be cured with appropriate treatment. Treatment options depend on a number of factors including patients' health and age, the location and size of the tumor, and the type of tumor. Treatment can include surgery, chemotherapy, or radiotherapy. Sites of tumors include the lungs, brain, bladder, breast, skin, prostate, and bowel.

3-SECOND DOSE
Cancer is a disease where abnormal cells reproduce uncontrollably—they can invade and destroy healthy tissues of the body.

3-MINUTE TREATMENT
Cancer typically begins in one part of the body, known as the primary cancer, before spreading to other areas. The process of spreading to other tissues is known as metastasis. Metastasis occurs when cells break away from a cancerous tumor and travel through the bloodstream or through lymph vessels to other areas of the body.

RELATED ENTRIES
See also
HUMAN GENOME PROJECT (HGP)
page 36

CANCER TREATMENTS
page 72

RADIOTHERAPIST
page 122

3-SECOND BIOGRAPHY
MARIE CURIE
1867–1934
Polish physicist and chemist who pioneered research on radioactivity, later useful for cancer treatment; she won the Nobel Prize for Chemistry in 1911

EXPERT
Gabrielle M. Finn

Cancer cells spread to and destroy healthy cells within the body. Marie Curie's research on radioactivity showed that radiation could be used to destroy cancer cells.

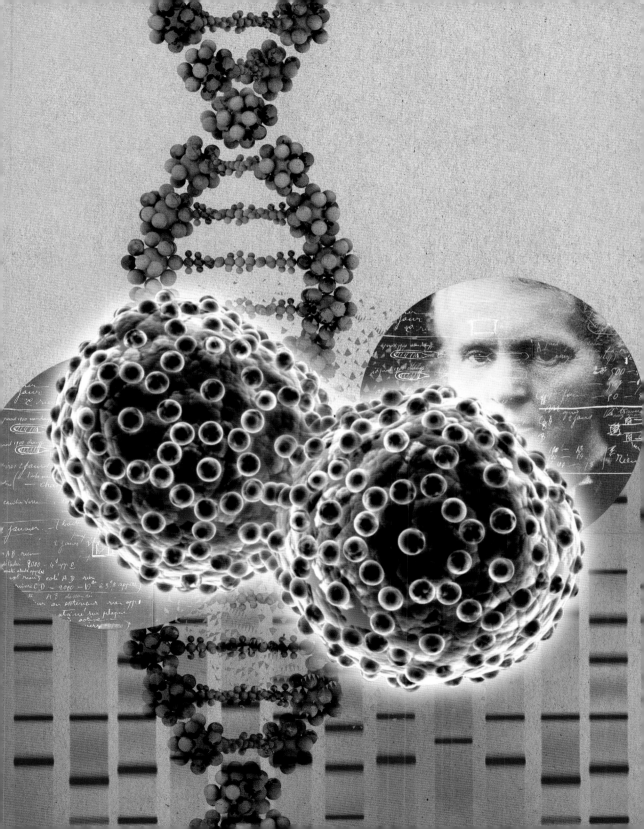

CYSTIC FIBROSIS (CF)

3-SECOND DOSE

Cystic fibrosis is an inherited (genetic) disease caused by a faulty gene, known as the CFTR gene, which is responsible for creating a protein that moves salt and water out of a cell.

3-MINUTE TREATMENT

Gene therapy is currently being trialed as a potential cure for cystic fibrosis. Researchers have been trialing insertion of a normal copy of the CFTR gene into affected cells. It is hoped that this will result in the production of functional CFTR in all target cells and thus restore functionality of the gene and protein in patients.

Cystic fibrosis is inherited from birth. If someone inherits the faulty gene from one parent then they may become a carrier, but if someone inherits the faulty gene from both parents then they will suffer from CF. Unlike many other diseases, CF cannot be passed on through body fluids. Newborn screening tests are available in most countries to identify those who have inherited the disease—testing requires a small blood sample, usually taken from the baby's heel. CF symptoms can differ immensely from patient to patient. The disease impacts on many systems of the body including the respiratory, digestive, and reproductive systems. Within the lungs and digestive tract, the genetic defect causes a build-up of thick mucus that makes breathing and digesting food very difficult. The mucus can trap particles, leading to the patient suffering from repeated infections. Malnutrition can lead to brittle bones, and reproductive organs become blocked by excessive mucus. There is no cure for CF, however life expectancy has increased significantly with modern treatments. Antibiotics are used to fight infection, while physiotherapy helps to mobilize mucus and prevent too much build-up. Some patients receive organ transplants in order to help prolong their lives. Historically, patients died in childhood but now life expectancy is into adulthood.

RELATED ENTRIES

See also
ORGAN DONATION
& TRANSPLANT
page 30

HUMAN GENOME PROJECT
(HGP)
page 36

ANTIBIOTICS
page 76

PHYSIOTHERAPIST
page 116

3-SECOND BIOGRAPHY
DOROTHY ANDERSEN
1901–63
American physician who first described cystic fibrosis

EXPERT
Gabrielle M. Finn

Cystic fibrosis is a genetic disease that causes a build-up of thick mucus in the lungs and digestive tract. If both parents carry the CF gene, there's a one in four chance of the child being affected.

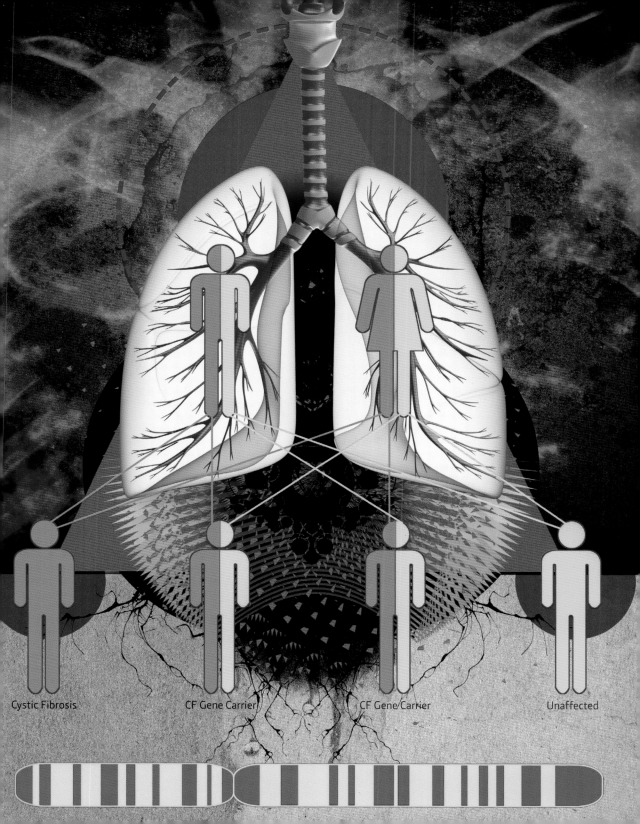

Cystic Fibrosis   CF Gene Carrier   CF Gene Carrier   Unaffected

EBOLA VIRUS DISEASE

3-SECOND DOSE

Ebola virus disease, also known as Ebola hemorrhagic fever or Ebola, is a disease transmitted to humans by the Ebola virus.

3-MINUTE TREATMENT

The first Ebola outbreak documented was in 1976 in Sudan and Zaire. Other outbreaks between 1976 and the present have often been focused around Africa. An outbreak first reported in West Africa in March 2014 caused at least 11,312 deaths.

The Ebola virus was identified in 1976. It causes an infectious illness that often proves fatal. Ebola is contracted if someone comes into contact with the body fluids (blood, urine, semen, and so on) or organs of an infected person. Once infected, patients typically develop symptoms including fever, headache, sore throat, intense muscle weakness, and joint and muscle pain. Vomiting, a rash, and diarrhea usually follow. Patients frequently experience bleeding; this can be both internal and external. Bleeding can be seen from the nose, mouth, and eyes, as well as within feces. The onset of symptoms can be sudden and typically starts between two and 21 days of becoming infected. People do not become infectious until they have developed symptoms. Ebola can be fatal. Death is usually associated with dehydration and low blood pressure from fluid loss. Patients may experience multiple organ failure. Ebola patients need to be kept in isolation due to the highly infectious nature of the disease. Treatment typically focuses on management of symptoms, for example rehydration, or palliative care for the dying. In 2015, a potential treatment known as ZMapp was tested. Early research results of animal trials showed promising reversal of advanced Ebola virus disease. A preventative Ebola vaccine has also been trialed in the UK and USA.

RELATED ENTRY

See also
IMMUNIZATION & VACCINATION
page 70

3-SECOND BIOGRAPHY

PETER PIOT
1949–
Belgian scientist who first discovered Ebola in 1976

EXPERT

Gabrielle M. Finn

There have been several outbreaks of Ebola in Africa. The virus causes a serious and highly infectious disease.

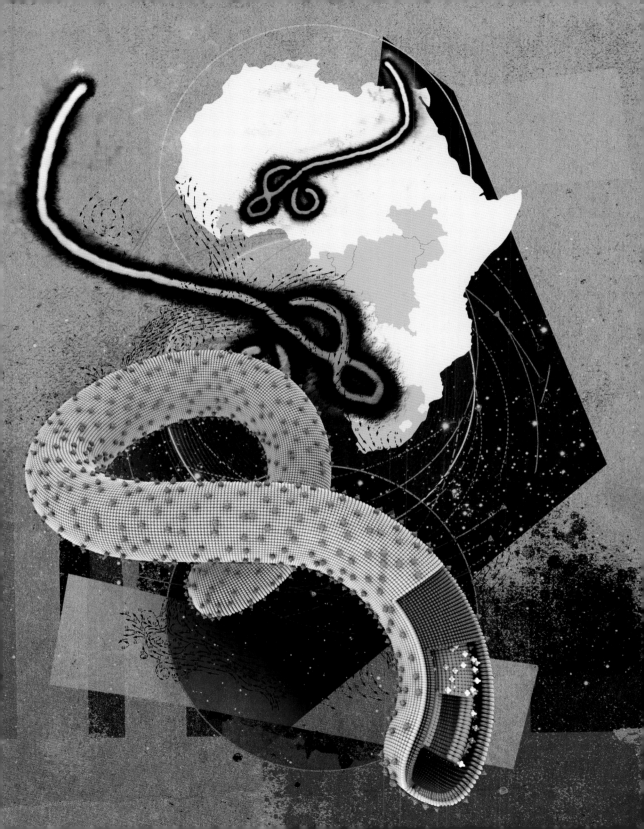

ROLES IN MEDICINE

ROLES IN MEDICINE
GLOSSARY

clinical technologist Also known as medical technologists, clinical technologists are responsible for maintaining, monitoring, and operating any instruments utilized within the hospital environment for treating and diagnosing patients.

forceps A pair of tweezers used in surgery or in a laboratory. Larger version with wide gripping paddles are used to assist with delivering a baby's head during childbirth.

geriatric A term relating to old people, most frequently used with regard to their health care, for example a geriatrician is a doctor who specializes in care of the elderly.

hydrotherapy Also known as water therapy, hydrotherapy is the use of water (hot, cold, steam, or ice) to relieve discomfort and promote mobility. Typically, hydrotherapy occurs in a large pool of water. Symptoms from conditions such as arthritis can be relieved using hydrotherapy.

manual therapy The use of skilled hand movements to manipulate tissues of the body to restore movement, alleviate pain, promote general health, or induce relaxation.

oncologist A doctor who treats cancer. Usually, an oncologist manages a patient's care and treatment once they have been diagnosed with cancer.

orthopedics The medical specialty concerned with the preservation, restoration and development of function of the musculoskeletal system, limbs and spine.

pediatrics A medical specialty that deals with the care of infants, children and adolescents. In the UK this is a hospital speciality. In other countries, such as the USA, pediatrics is also available within primary care.

primary care Health care provided in the community for patients making an initial approach to a medical practitioner or clinic for advice or treatment. Family physicians/ family doctors are major providers of primary care.

radiation Energy in the form of a wave or particle that comes from a source and travels through some material or through space. Light, heat, and sound are types of radiation.

soft tissue Tissues of the body such as tendons, ligaments, skin, fat, connective tissue, muscles, nerves, and blood vessels.

PHYSIOTHERAPIST

RELATED ENTRIES
See also
ARTIFICIAL LIMBS
page 62

NURSE
page 118

DOCTOR
page 120

EXPERT
Larissa Nelson

3-SECOND DOSE
Physiotherapists aim to restore their patients' movement and function through manual therapy, education, and advice.

3-MINUTE TREATMENT
Modern physiotherapists can work independently or together with other health care professionals; however, a patient does not need a referral from a doctor in order to see a physiotherapist. To qualify as a physiotherapist, university-level education is required. In most countries physiotherapists must be registered with a licensing body in order to practice. Chartered physiotherapists must also provide evidence that they are updating their skills and knowledge annually and that they are committed to continuing professional development.

Physiotherapy techniques date as far back as 460 BCE when early physicians such as Hippocrates practiced elements of manual therapy. The profession, however, started to become recognized in the 1800s when physiotherapists were able to become officially registered in some countries. Physiotherapists are trained in assessing, diagnosing, treating, and preventing a wide range of health care issues using evidence-based techniques, helping people of all ages who have been affected by injury, illness, or disability. They often use movement and manual therapy to deal with conditions associated with different systems of the body including the musculoskeletal system (bones, joints, and soft tissues), the neuromuscular system (the brain and nervous system), the cardiovascular system (the heart and blood circulation), and the respiratory system. Conditions that physiotherapists commonly treat include asthma, back pain, cerebral palsy, osteoporosis, and chronic obstructive pulmonary disease. Physiotherapists help their patients recover from difficulties that may have been present from birth, acquired through accident or injury, or developed over time. Examples of treatment methods that physiotherapists commonly use include soft tissue mobilization, hydrotherapy, and joint manipulation.

Physiotherapists use a range of therapies to treat different conditions and also develop exercise programs for their patients to improve mobility and to strengthen or retrain muscles.

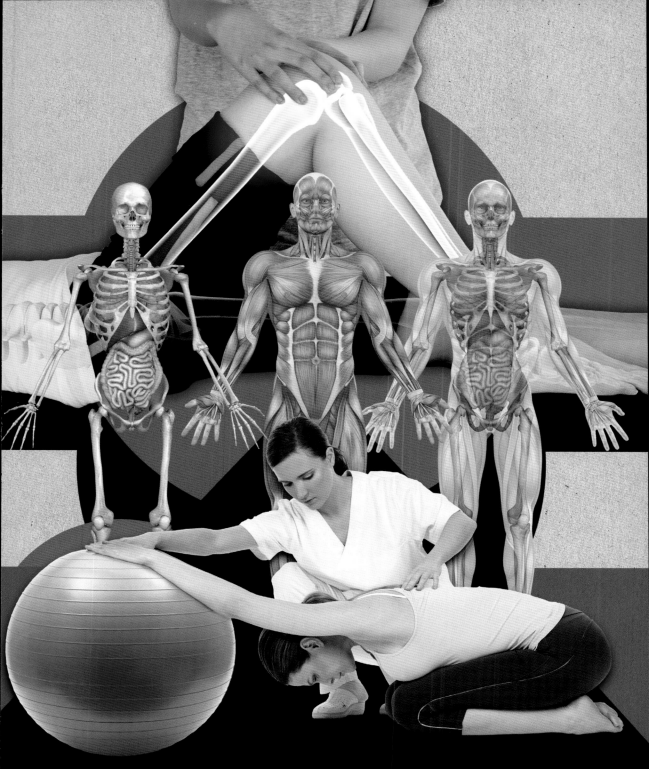

NURSE

3-SECOND DOSE

A nurse is a health care professional whose aim is to ensure quality care of individuals of all ages, families, groups, and communities.

3-MINUTE TREATMENT

The role of nurses can be very diverse. In addition to providing the best possible care for their patients, they may also be involved in the promotion of health and safe environments and the prevention of illness. They may act as advocates or be involved in reshaping health policies. More experienced nurses also have the potential to work in research or in education.

Nurses combine the art of caring with scientific knowledge and clinical skills. They are involved in assisting people in performing activities that contribute to health or recovery, and are trained in dealing with individuals who are disabled or sick. Nurses will often work in a team with other health professionals, but are usually the main point of contact for patients. Nurses' roles range greatly depending on their interests and the health setting in which they work. For example, a nurse working in an emergency department within a hospital will often be faced with a stressful and fast-paced environment where stabilizing patients may be one of their first priorities. A contrasting example is a learning disability nurse whose aim is to improve the well-being and social inclusion of their patients in a comfortable setting. Nurses must undergo formal university-level education and training before they are able to register. Although there are many fields, the four main specialist areas are adult nursing, children's nursing, learning disability nursing, and mental health nursing. Examples of settings that nurses work in include hospitals, clinics, and medical centers, as well as in schools, camps, private and retirement homes, prisons, and even on cruise ships.

RELATED ENTRIES

See also
FLORENCE NIGHTINGALE
page 124

PHYSICIAN ASSISTANT (PA)
page 126

MIDWIFE
page 130

3-SECOND BIOGRAPHIES

CLAIRE BERTSCHINGER
1960–
Anglo-Swiss nurse who became renowned for her work with the International Red Cross dealing with famine in Ethiopia in the 1980s; she won the Florence Nightingale Medal in 1991

WILLIAM POOLEY
1985–
British nurse who contracted Ebola while working in West Africa to combat the outbreak; he was awarded an MBE for his services

EXPERT

Larissa Nelson

Assisting both patients and professionals, nurses are employed in a wide range of health care settings.

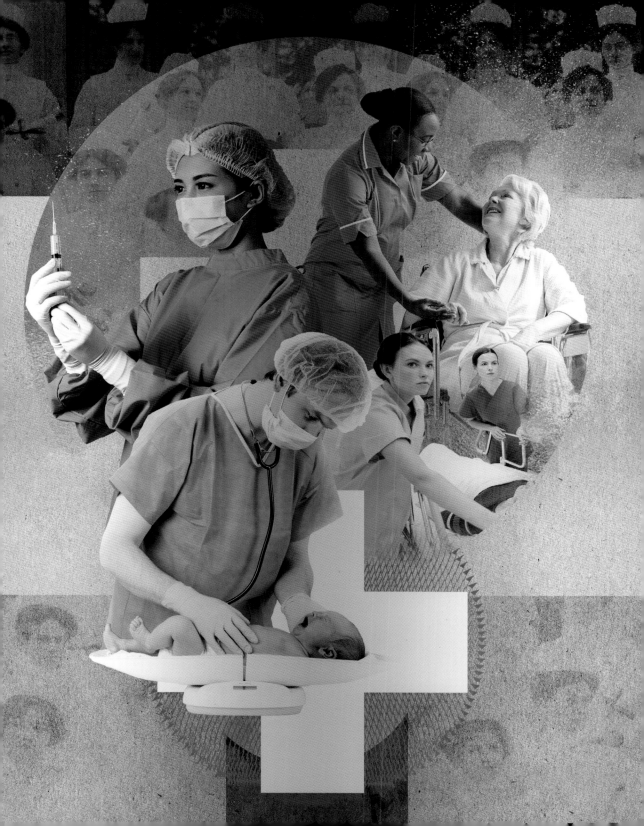

DOCTOR

Medical doctors, sometimes referred to as physicians or medical practitioners, are involved in examining, diagnosing, and treating patients who arrive with illness, disease, injuries, pain, or other conditions. Some would say that together with nurses, they form the backbone of health care systems. Doctors usually work in a team with several other health care professionals, and apply their scientific knowledge and clinical judgement to ensure that the most effective patient care is achieved. They must have the ability to assimilate new knowledge critically, be able to make decisions efficiently, and be capable of dealing with uncertainty and complexity. Doctors usually work in hospitals or clinics, and their daily activities vary depending on the area of medicine they have chosen to specialize in. Some of the most common specialties within a hospital are emergency medicine, general surgery, trauma, orthopedics, pediatrics, and psychiatry. Family doctors' roles can vary greatly; however, they usually provide primary and continuing medical care for patients in the community. In some countries they may also travel to rural areas to provide care to other communities. Doctors prescribe medication and develop treatment plans that may involve referring patients to specialists for more specific assessments.

3-SECOND DOSE
Doctors are medically trained health professionals who aim to promote, maintain, and restore health in their patients.

3-MINUTE TREATMENT
A university degree and extensive clinical training are prerequisites to becoming a doctor. That said, it is not all about being intellectually capable. Doctors require many qualities in order to provide the best possible care to their patients, which include being committed, caring, and compassionate. Doctors need to act with integrity and respect, and must deal confidentially with their patients. Competence and concern for people are also imperative to being a good doctor.

RELATED ENTRIES
See also
JOSEPH LISTER
page 38

NURSE
page 118

PHYSICIAN ASSISTANT (PA)
page 126

3-SECOND BIOGRAPHY
EDWARD JENNER
1749–1823
English doctor who discovered the vaccine for smallpox; his work is said to have saved more lives than the work of any other individual

EXPERT
Larissa Nelson

Whether specialist or family doctor, doctors are involved with examining, diagnosing, and treating patients.

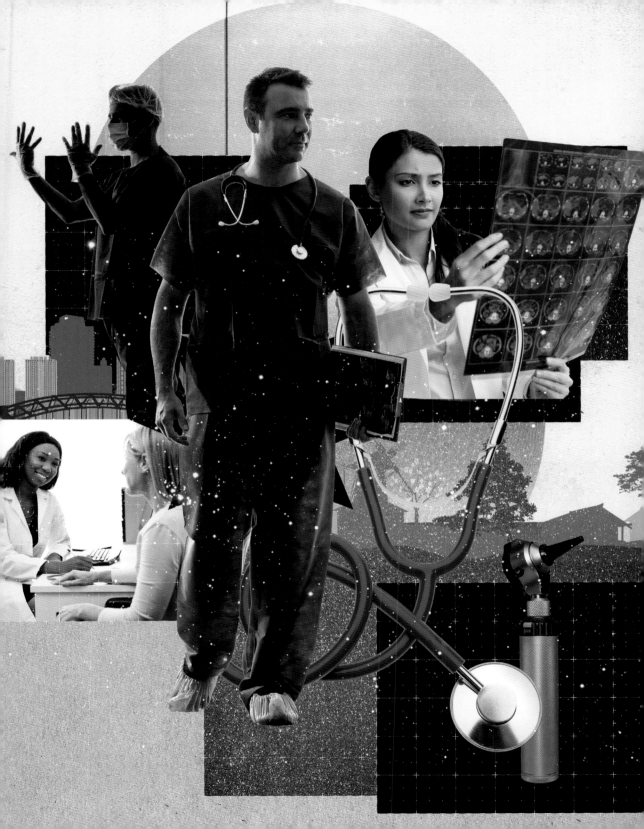

RADIOTHERAPIST

Radiotherapists work within a
multidisciplinary team together with clinical
oncologists, clinical technologists, and support
staff to provide radiation treatment to patients.
Radiotherapists are trained in areas of oncology
and psychosocial issues surrounding cancer care,
as radiotherapy is commonly used as part of a
treatment plan for cancer sufferers. Radiotherapy
can also be used to treat other conditions such
as non-cancerous tumors and thyroid disease.
The role of the radiotherapist is to calculate
appropriate radiation doses and administer
the treatment using innovative technologies. As
new techniques and technologies are constantly
emerging, radiotherapists need to be aware
of advances in their field. Radiotherapy can
be administered externally (outside the body) or
internally (inside the body). External radiotherapy
focuses the radiation beams onto a specific
target area, damaging the DNA of cells and
causing them to die. In addition to damaging
the target cancer cells, nearby healthy cells are
also affected. Internal radiotherapy involves
inserting a small piece of radioactive material
inside the body near the target destination.
Radiotherapists are responsible for the precision
and accuracy of the treatment. They are also
responsible for assessing and evaluating the
patient's condition throughout the process.

3-SECOND DOSE
A radiotherapist is a
healthcare professional
who plans and administers
treatments using
high-energy radiation.

3-MINUTE TREATMENT
Radiotherapists must
undergo university-level
education in order
to qualify, and can be
involved in clinical practice
at all levels ranging from
assistant to service
manager. They may also
choose to specialize in
specific technologies,
or in treating certain
cancers or patient
groups. Radiotherapists
are often involved in
clinical research evaluating
technologies or treatments
to ensure that evidence-
based practice is achieved.

RELATED ENTRIES
See also
MAGNETIC RESONANCE
IMAGING (MRI)
page 54

CANCER TREATMENTS
page 72

CANCER
page 106

3-SECOND BIOGRAPHY
LEOPOLD FREUND
1868–1943
Professor of radiology at the
Medical University of Vienna,
Austria; he is as considered as
the founder of radiotherapy
and was one of the first known
to have used radiation for
therapeutic purposes

EXPERT
Larissa Nelson

*Radiotherapists devise
and apply treatment
plans—most commonly
radiation treatments
for cancer patients—
using high-energy
radiation technology.*

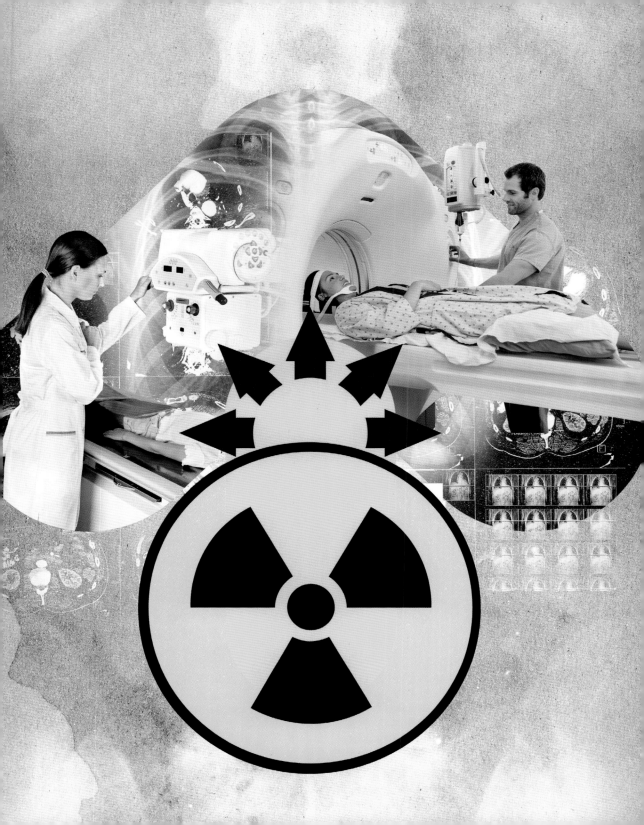

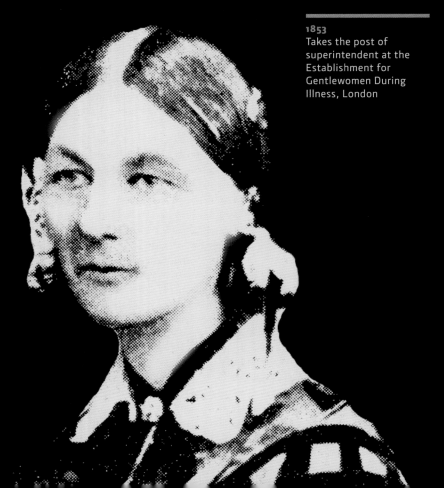

1820
Born in Florence,
Italy, after which she
was named

1837
While at the family
home at Embley Park,
Hampshire, experiences
her first "call from God,"
prompting a desire to
go into nursing

1847
Meets Sidney Herbert,
who would become
Secretary of War during
the Crimean War and
who was instrumental
in enacting many of
her reforms

1851
Undertakes four months
of medical training in
Kaiserswerth, Germany

1853
Takes the post of
superintendent at the
Establishment for
Gentlewomen During
Illness, London

1854
Arrives at Selimiye
Barracks in Scutari,
Turkey, with a team
of volunteer nurses
and Catholic nuns to
tend to the wounded
British soldiers of the
Crimean War

1858
Elected a member of the
Royal Statistical Society,
its first female member

1859
Publishes *Notes on
Nursing*

1860
Establishment of the
Nightingale Training
School for Nurses at
St. Thomas' Hospital,
London

1910
Dies in her sleep at
her house in South
Street, Mayfair, London

FLORENCE NIGHTINGALE

Forever remembered as "The Lady with the Lamp," Florence Nightingale remains the archetype of the caring, compassionate nurse in the minds of many people. Yet, her upper-class background made her a very unlikely nurse in the nineteenth century. The Nightingale family was opposed to Florence taking up nursing, preferring her to become a wife and mother as expected of women of her status. However, she rebelled against her parents' wishes and in 1851 undertook four months of training in Kaiserswerth, Germany. Two years later, she returned to London to take the position of superintendent in the Establishment for Gentlewomen During Illness.

Nightingale's fame as a nurse began during her time at the hospital in Scutari (part of modern-day Istanbul) during the Crimean War. Following reports in the British press of the poor conditions of the military hospitals, she traveled there with a team of nurses to tend to the wounded soldiers. On arrival she was horrified at the lack of hygiene, the scarcity of medicines, and overcrowding. Such were the insanitary conditions that ten times as many patients were dying of infection as of battle wounds. She immediately set to work implementing hygienic practices (such as handwashing), acquiring clean clothing and bed linen, and reorganizing the kitchen and laundries. In doing so, Nightingale drastically reduced the death rates from 42 percent to 2 percent.

Back in England, Nightingale continued to campaign for better sanitation and ventilation in army hospitals and barracks, and was instrumental in the founding of the Royal Army Medical College, before turning her attention to hospital reform more generally, improving conditions in workhouses and infirmaries. Using funds donated by the public during her time in the Crimea, the Nightingale Training School for Nurses was founded in 1860 at St. Thomas' Hospital, London.

Much of Nightingale's success was possible because of her pioneering use of the graphical presentation of statistics. She developed a form of pie chart now known as the polar area diagram to display seasonal variations in causes of mortality in the Scutari hospital. These diagrams helped members of parliament and civil servants understand the impact of the insanitary conditions and the positive effects of her reforms.

The achievements of Florence Nightingale in the fields of medical care and statistics have ensured her continued legacy. Her commitment to compassion and patient care set the standards for the modern profession of nursing which are still upheld today.

Philip Cox

PHYSICIAN ASSISTANT (PA)

RELATED ENTRY
See also
DOCTOR
page 120

3-SECOND DOSE
A physician assistant is a health care professional whose role is to support doctors in the diagnosis and management of patients.

3-MINUTE TREATMENT
University-level academic attainment, as well as experience in the health care industry, are normally prerequisites to PA training. The course itself usually consists of extensive theoretical and practical clinical training over a two- to three-year period. The first PA graduates were from Duke University, North Carolina in 1967. Once qualified, PAs are required to show yearly evidence of continuing professional development, and must take periodic recertification exams in order to remain certified.

Physician assistant (USA) and physician associate (UK) are interchangeable terms for related roles. Many other countries have similar roles within their medical models that fall under different job titles. The role of a physician assistant was first developed in the USA in the 1960s to address the shortage of medical providers. Today, they are nationally certified and state licensed to practice, with over 100,000 across the USA. In the UK, the role is a relatively new health care profession and in 2012 there was a drive to change the name from assistant to associate. In addition to the USA and the UK, PA initiatives also exist in other countries including Australia, Canada, and the Netherlands. PAs can practice in both primary care and other medical specialities, and they have direct contact with patients. They are trained to perform tasks including taking medical histories, performing examinations, diagnosing and treating illnesses, analyzing test results, and developing treatment plans. In some places they can also assist in surgery. In the USA, PAs are authorized to prescribe medication. PAs work under the direct supervision of a doctor in order to help deliver high-quality medical care, usually in adult medical specialties. Settings include family doctors' offices and clinics, hospital inpatient wards, geriatric wards, and accident and emergency units.

3-SECOND BIOGRAPHY
EUGENE ANSON STEAD
1908–2005
American medical educator and founder of the Physician Assistant profession, graduating the first class of PAs in 1967

EXPERT
Larissa Nelson

Physician assistants work in a variety of medical settings providing clinical support for doctors.

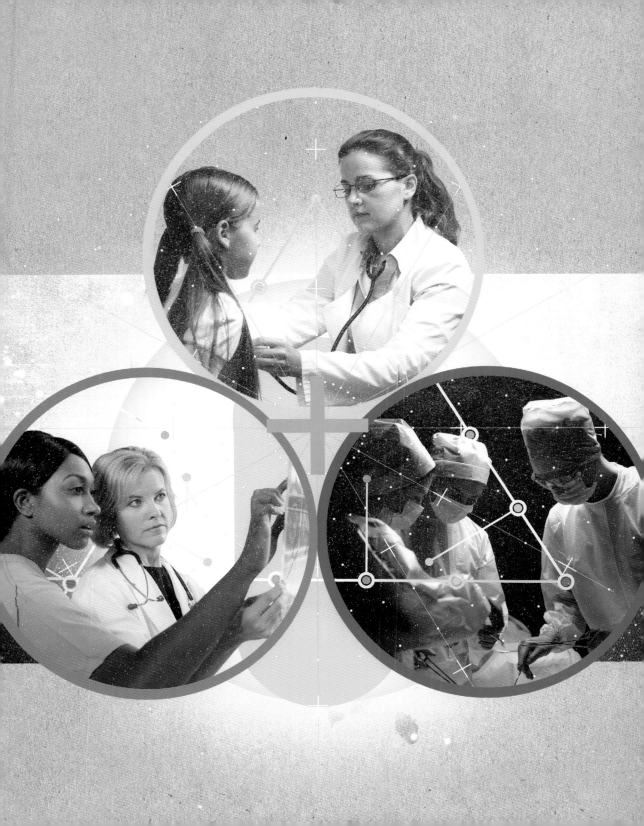

PHARMACIST

3-SECOND DOSE

Pharmacists are health care professionals who are experts in the field of drugs and medicines, focusing on safe and effective use of medication.

3-MINUTE TREATMENT

In most countries, pharmacists are required to undergo university-level education and a period of pre-registration training before they are able to fully qualify. They need to understand the biochemical mechanisms and actions of drugs and their interactions. In addition to this sound scientific understanding, pharmacists also require excellent communication and interpersonal skills, as well as accuracy and meticulous attention to detail because they are legally responsible for any dispensing errors.

Pharmacists are directly involved in patient care and are often the first point of contact for people with health enquiries. They follow legal and ethical guidelines to ensure that patients receive informed advice on type, dose, and appropriate form of medication. Most pharmacists are community based in pharmacies, supermarkets, and local healthcare centers. A smaller proportion are hospital based where they work closely with medical and nursing staff. In addition to providing advice, community pharmacists prepare and dispense prescription medication, and also sell non-prescription medication. They will ask questions to ensure that the medication they are recommending is compatible with other treatments the patient may be undergoing. The pharmacist will also inform patients about possible side effects and precautions that should be taken. Some community pharmacists may offer specialist health care checks, clinics, or programs. Hospital pharmacists are often involved in taking patient drug histories and in discussing treatment options with doctors, other pharmacists, the patients, and their relatives. Some hospital-based pharmacists are qualified to prescribe certain medication themselves. More experienced pharmacists may also be involved in research, teaching, or supervising less experienced staff.

RELATED ENTRIES
See also
NURSE
page 118

DOCTOR
page 120

3-SECOND BIOGRAPHIES
FRIEDRICH SERTÜRNER
1783–1841
German pharmacist who discovered morphine in 1804; his research into the effects of morphine helped lead to its use in pain relief today

JOHN PEMBERTON
1831–88
American pharmacist best known for creating Coca-Cola; it was initially invented as a drink containing alcohol that was used to counteract his addiction to morphine

EXPERT
Larissa Nelson

Pharmacists use their knowledge of medications to complete prescriptions and advise patients.

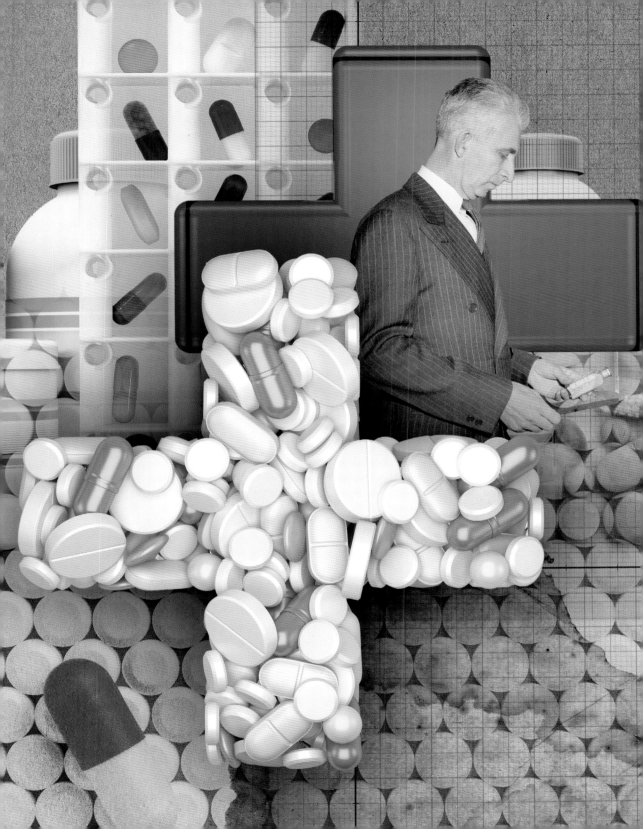

MIDWIFE

Midwifery is a health profession

that supports pregnant women and their families through all aspects relating to normal childbirth. Where problems arise, they need to be able to detect them and refer them to doctors or other specialized individuals. Midwives can work in hospitals, birth centers, or be community based where they make home visits or run clinics. During labor and childbirth, midwives provide information and support to expecting parents and birth partners, while also monitoring the health of the mother and baby. They take measures to avoid unnecessary interference in the progression of normal labor and childbirth. If the baby is distressed or the mother can't push any more, a midwife may recommend an assisted birth in which forceps or a vacuum extractor may be used, particularly in developed countries. Historically, midwives were women who acquired their skills as apprentices to older women who were experienced in giving birth themselves. Between the eighteenth and nineteenth centuries, however, there was a change in opinion and many believed that male physicians were safer, and that women midwives were incompetent and ignorant. In the nineteenth century, the status of female midwives was reinstated, although there was some resistance to recognizing midwifery as a profession in case it affected doctors' practices.

3-SECOND DOSE
A midwife is someone who provides support and care for women during pregnancy, childbirth, and for a period following the birth of a baby.

3-MINUTE TREATMENT
Certified nurse-midwives are now recognized as highly trained and specialized professionals. They must be able to remain calm and alert in stressful situations, while treating people with kindness, respect, and compassion. Midwives receive theoretical and practical training through approved university degree courses covering aspects of biological sciences, sociology, psychology, as well as professional practice. In many countries apprenticeships are no longer recognized as formal training, however alternative routes into midwifery do exist.

RELATED ENTRIES
See also
ULTRASOUND
page 56

DOCTOR
page 120

3-SECOND BIOGRAPHIES
JANE SHARP
1641–71
The first English midwife to publish a book on midwifery; *The Midwives Book*; or, *The Whole Art of Midwifery Discovered* became one of the best-known English textbooks on midwifery

INA MAY GASKIN
1940–
Has been described as America's leading midwife; in 1971 she founded one of the first out-of-hospital birth centers in Tennessee called the The Farm Midwifery Center and has won several awards in recognition of her work

EXPERT
Larissa Nelson

Midwives provide information and support to parents during pregnancy and labor.

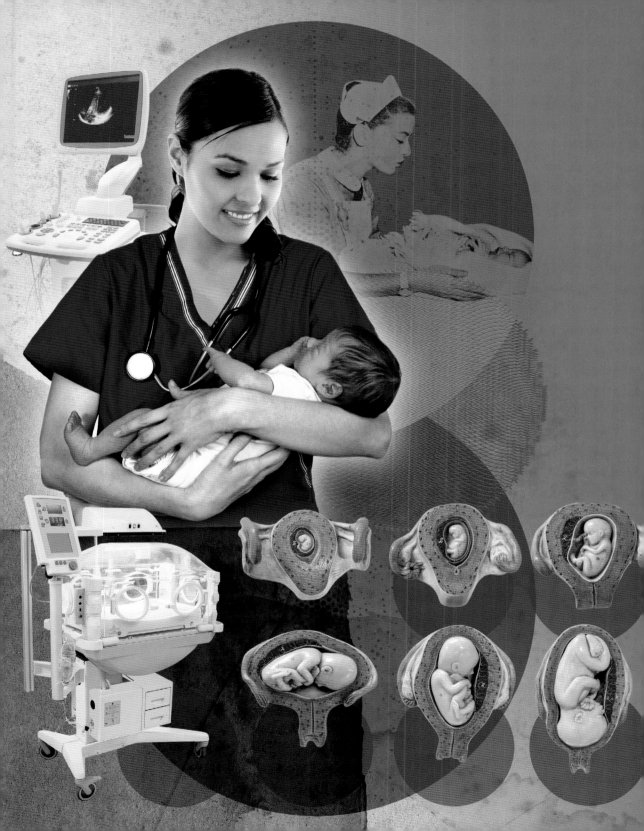

DRUGS

anabolic hormone A chemical that promotes cell growth by building up molecules into something new once they've been broken down. Many anabolic hormones are naturally secreted by the body, for example insulin and testosterone.

anti-inflammatory Typically refers to the property of a drug or treatment that reduces inflammation or swelling.

antipyretic analgesic Antipyretics are substances that reduce fever. They cause the brain to override an increase in body temperature. An analgesic is a medicine that takes away physical pain.

beta cells A type of cell found in the pancreas. They produce, store, and release the hormone insulin.

cannabinoids Active chemical compounds found in cannabis that interact with the cannabinoid receptors in the brain.

cannabinoid receptors These are located in the brain. They form part of the endocannabinoid system, which is involved in a variety of physiological processes including appetite, pain-sensation, mood, and memory.

cognitive behavioral therapy (CBT) A form of psychotherapy. It is often referred to as "talking therapy" and is used for a number of mental disorders. It works to change unhelpful thinking and behavior.

dopamine A chemical messenger (neurotransmitter) that helps control the brain's reward and pleasure centers. It has a role in helping regulate movement and emotional responses.

gastric acid The acid within the stomach that aids digestion.

intravenous The term for when a liquid substance is infused or injected directly into a vein.

lipids Molecules that have a function in storing energy, signaling, and acting as structural components of cell membranes. Lipids include fats, fat-soluble vitamins, hormones, oils, and waxes.

noradrenaline (NA) Also called norepinephrine (NE), NA is a hormone and neurotransmitter (chemical messenger) found naturally within the body. It is often referred to as a "fight or flight" chemical, as it is responsible for the body's reaction to stressful situations. It is given by injection to treat life-threatening drops in blood pressure (hypotension).

pathway A biological pathway is a sequence of actions between molecules in a cell that leads to a certain product or a change in a cell. Pathways can generate the creation of new molecules or turn genes on and off.

pharmacology The study of the actions of drugs. Pharmacologists work to understand the actions, sources, and properties of medications.

psychoactive drugs Chemical substances that change brain function. Their actions can lead to alterations in mood, perception, or consciousness.

Reye's syndrome A condition that causes swelling in the liver and brain. It most commonly affects children and teenagers recovering from viral infections such as chickenpox or flu. It is rare but very serious.

serotonin A neurotransmitter (chemical messenger). It can affect the functioning of the cardiovascular system, muscles, and various elements in the endocrine (glands) system.

subcutaneous The term for when a liquid substance is infused or injected into the tissue layer beneath the skin.

thrombin An enzyme in blood plasma that causes the clotting of blood by converting fibrinogen (a protein) into fibrin (a protein which forms the blood clot).

tricyclics antidepressants (TCAs) A class of antidepressants used extensively for treatment of depression. They prevent nerve cells from reabsorbing chemical messengers, such as noradrenaline and serotonin, and thereby prolong the mood-elevating effect of noradrenaline and serotonin to help relieve depression.

vitamin K A group of compounds that have a key role in the formation of the factors that enable blood to clot.

ACETAMINOPHEN

Acetaminophen, or paracetamol as it is also known, is a common over-the-counter treatment for mild to moderate pain and fevers. It is derived from acetanilide and phenacetin, earlier antipyretic analgesics, which had significant side effects limiting their use. Acetaminophen was first used in the USA in the 1950s and can now be found in most households' medicine cabinets. Despite its widespread use, its mechanism of action is not clearly understood. It affects cyclooxygenase enzymes, which are critical in the formation of prostaglandins, chemicals which are responsible, in part, for both pain and fever. This is a common pathway shared with other simple pain killers such as aspirin. An active metabolite of acetaminophen may also affect central cannabinoid receptors, which are involved in the sensation of pain. Acetaminophen can be administered both orally and parenterally (by injection) and comes in many different forms including tablets, capsules, liquid suspensions, and suppositories. Adults and children can take acetaminophen safely, with the maximum adult daily dose being 4 grams. This dose is important as even slight increases may lead to toxicity and liver failure. This is especially an issue with acetaminophen overdoses, which are common. However, the medication N-acetylcysteine administered urgently and intravenously can prevent significant complications.

3-SECOND DOSE

Acetaminophen is a safe and widely used medication for the management of both pain and fevers, which can cause significant problems in overdose.

3-MINUTE TREATMENT

Acetaminophen was created accidently by Harmon Morse, an American chemist, in 1878. However, use of acetaminophen was widespread from the 1950s and was assisted by its favorable side-effect profile compared to other analgesics such as aspirin, which caused peptic ulcers. The revelation that aspirin use in children was associated with Reye's syndrome (early 1980s) led to acetaminophen becoming the first choice antipyretic analgesic not only in children but for all ages.

RELATED ENTRIES

See also
PROTON PUMP INHIBITORS (PPI)
page 146

CANNABIS
page 150

3-SECOND BIOGRAPHIES

HARMON NORTHROP MORSE
1848–1920
American chemist and professor at Johns Hopkins University, who was the first to synthesize acetaminophen

JULIUS AXELROD
1912–2004
American biochemist who first used acetaminophen, as an analgesic, in human studies

EXPERT

Martin Veysey

Acetaminophen is one of the most widely used medications. It is used to relieve mild pain and manage fevers.

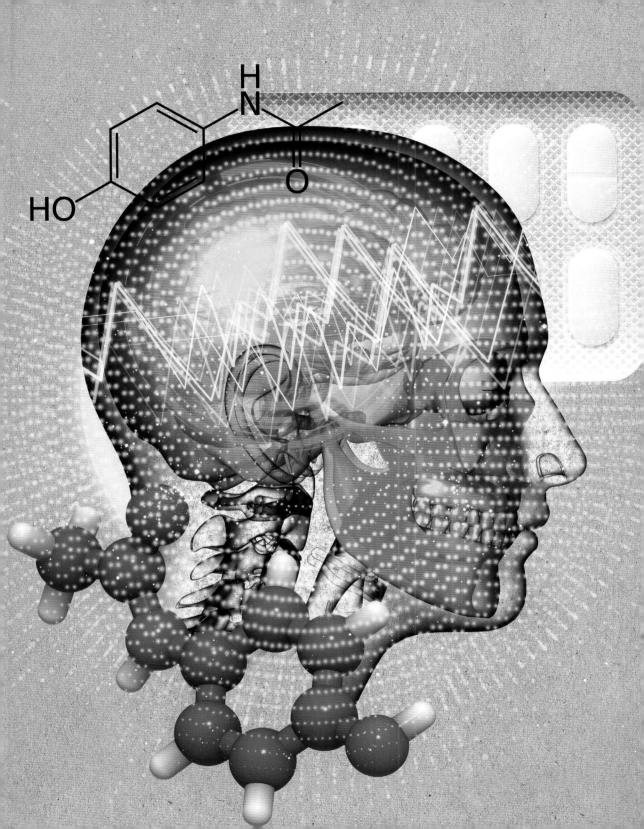

ANTIDEPRESSANTS

3-SECOND DOSE
Antidepressants,
which modulate
neurotransmitters, are
used effectively to treat
moderate to severe
depression and a number
of other psychiatric
conditions.

3-MINUTE TREATMENT
The first antidepressant
drugs were discovered
in the 1950s when a
developmental treatment
for tuberculosis was noted
to make patients more
cheerful. There are also
a number of herbal
treatments that claim
antidepressant properties.
Hypericum, which contains
St. John's wort, is one of
these. However, there are
limited data on its efficacy
and preparations may vary.
Another possible treatment
for depression is cognitive
behavioral therapy.

More than 120 million people

worldwide suffer from depression and a significant number of them take antidepressant medications as part of their treatment. There are over 30 antidepressant medications in five classes. These include tricyclics (for example, amitriptyline), monoamine oxidase inhibitors (for example, phenelzine), selective serotonin re-uptake inhibitors (for example, fluoxetine), serotonin and noradrenaline re-uptake inhibitors (for example, venlaflaxine), and noradrenaline and specific serotoninergic antidepressants (for example, mirtazapine). The drugs work by normalizing chemicals in the brain, known as neurotransmitters. The neurotransmitters serotonin, noradrenaline, and dopamine are all thought to be chemicals important in controlling an individual's mood. The choice of medication usually depends on the clinical presentation of the patient, because each drug has slightly different effects. All the medications are effective in up to 60 percent of patients. The newer medications are often chosen because they have fewer side effects and are safer in overdoses. The side effects are specific to each medication, but include headaches, nausea, dry mouth, constipation, night sweats, and agitation. Patients normally need to take the medication regularly for three to four weeks for the optimal effect and will usually continue taking them for up to one year.

RELATED ENTRY
See also
PSYCHOTHERAPY
page 86

3-SECOND BIOGRAPHY
ROLAND KUHN
1951–2005
Swiss psychiatrist and
psychopharmacologist who
discovered that imipramine has
antidepressant properties

EXPERT
Martin Veysey

*Antidepressants
normalize the
neurotransmitters that
control mood. As well
as moderate to severe
depression, they can
be used to treat severe
anxiety and panic
disorders, obsessive
compulsive disorder,
chronic pain, and
post-traumatic
stress disorder.*

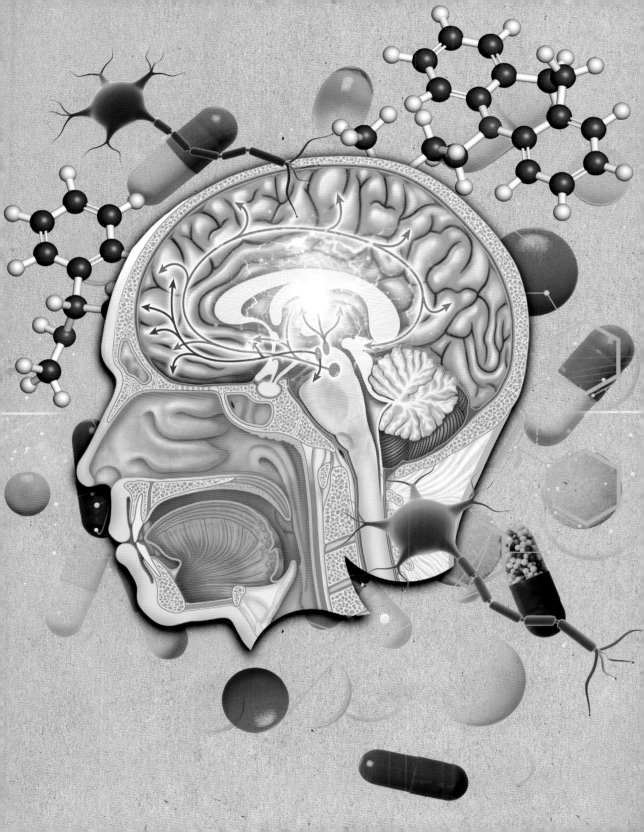

INSULIN

3-SECOND DOSE
Insulin is a hormone
produced by the pancreas
that controls blood sugar
levels, a deficiency of
which causes diabetes.

3-MINUTE TREATMENT
Another way for patients
with diabetes to receive
insulin is for them to
undergo a pancreas
transplant, in which a
healthy pancreas from
a donor is surgically
implanted in the abdominal
cavity. Insulin not only
controls blood sugar levels
but also a number of other
key metabolic processes.
It promotes synthesis of
fatty acids in the liver and
inhibits breakdown of fat
in adipose (fatty) tissue.
Insulin also stimulates the
uptake of amino acids.

Insulin is an anabolic hormone
produced by the beta cells of the pancreas.
While scientists in the nineteenth and early
twentieth centuries were able to show that
extracts from the pancreas lowered blood
sugars in animal models, it was not until 1921
that Dr. Frederick Banting and Charles H. Best
discovered that this effect was due to insulin.
Insulin maintains blood sugar or glucose levels
and prevents them from going too high
(hyperglycemia) or too low (hypoglycemia).
Insulin enables the body to absorb glucose,
transport it around the body and store it,
especially in the liver. If an individual does not
produce insulin, or is resistant to its effects,
they will develop diabetes, Type 1 or Type 2
respectively. Artificial insulin therapy was first
attempted one year after the discovery of
insulin. Initially, insulin treatments were derived
from cow (bovine) or pig (porcine) pancreas,
but these often caused immune reactions and
so recombinant DNA human insulin (made
by inserting the human gene for insulin into a
bacterium's genome) was developed and is now
widely used. There are four types of synthetic
insulin depending on their onset and duration
of action: rapid or short acting, intermediate
acting, long acting, and combinations of the
types. Patients administer the insulin by
subcutaneous injection with syringes, pens,
or a pump.

RELATED ENTRY
See also
DIABETES MELLITUS
page 96

3-SECOND BIOGRAPHIES
PAUL LANGERHANS
1847–88
German pathologist who
discovered and gave his name
to the pancreatic cells (Islets
of Langerhans) that produce
insulin

FREDERICK BANTING
& CHARLES H. BEST
1891–1941 & 1899–1978
Canadian doctor (Banting) and
his medical student (Best) who
discovered insulin

FREDERICK SANGER
1918–2013
British biochemist awarded a
Nobel Prize in Chemistry for his
work on the structure of insulin

EXPERT
Martin Veysey

*There are a variety
of insulin treatments
available for individuals
who either do not
produce insulin or are
resistant to its effects.*

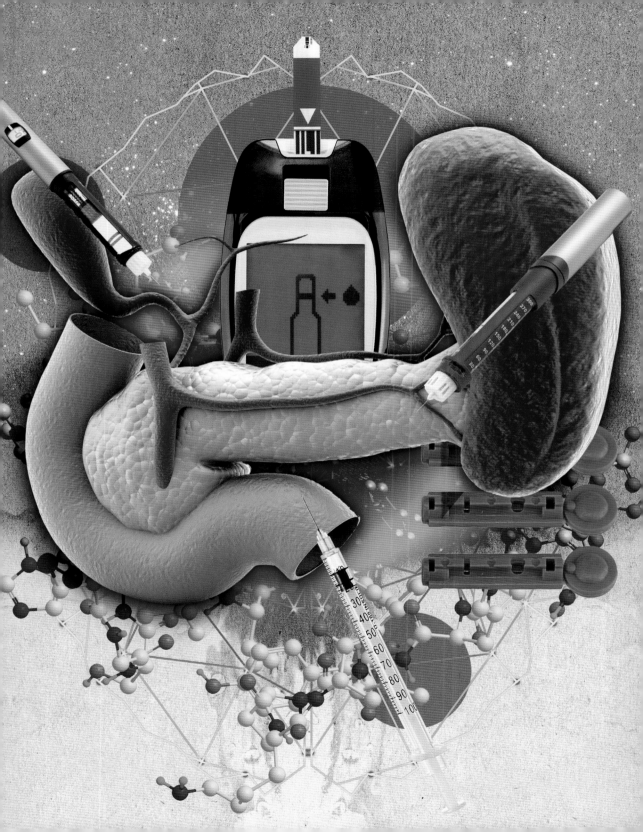

STATINS

3-SECOND DOSE
Statins are a class of drugs that significantly reduce blood levels of cholesterol and reduce the risk of cardiovascular disease.

3-MINUTE TREATMENT
Statins were originally derived from fungal specimens by Professor Akira Endo, who was trying to develop new antibiotic agents. However, what he found was a number of chemicals that stopped bacteria growing by blocking a key enzyme in the production of cholesterol within their cells. The first commercially available statin was lovastatin, but another, atorvastatin, is currently one of the best-selling pharmaceuticals of all time.

Statins, a group of medications that inhibit a key step in the synthesis of cholesterol within the body, inhibit an enzyme called hydroxymethylglutaryl CoA (HMG-CoA) reductase. This leads to a significant reduction in cholesterol levels in the blood as well as other impacts on an individual's lipid profile. High cholesterol levels, especially the low density lipoprotein (LDL) type of cholesterol, are associated with an increased risk of cardiovascular disease and reducing them can lead to significant reductions in both heart attacks and deaths. There is now good evidence for treating patients with increased risk but no evidence of cardiovascular disease (primary prevention), and those with early stage cardiovascular disease (secondary prevention). There are seven different commercially available statins: atorvastatin, fluvastatin, lovastatin, pitavastatin, pravastatin, rosuvastatin, and simvastatin. These medications have variations in their absorption and metabolism leading to differences in both potency and side effects. They can be used alone or in combination with other lipid-lowering agents. Side effects of statins include muscle pain and damage, an increased risk of Type 2 diabetes mellitus, and abnormalities in liver function tests. These should be monitored during treatment. In addition to taking medication, patients should consider making healthy lifestyle changes.

RELATED ENTRIES
See also
ANTIBIOTICS
page 76

DIABETES MELLITUS
page 96

VASCULAR DISEASE
page 98

3-SECOND BIOGRAPHIES
AKIRA ENDO
1933–
Japanese biochemist who conducted the initial work on isolating HMG-CoA reductase from fungi

JOSEPH GOLDSTEIN & MICHAEL BROWN
1940– & 1941–
American geneticists who won a Nobel prize for their work on cholesterol metabolism, which led to the development of statins

EXPERT
Martin Veysey

Statins inhibit the synthesis of cholesterol, reducing the risk of cardiovascular disease.

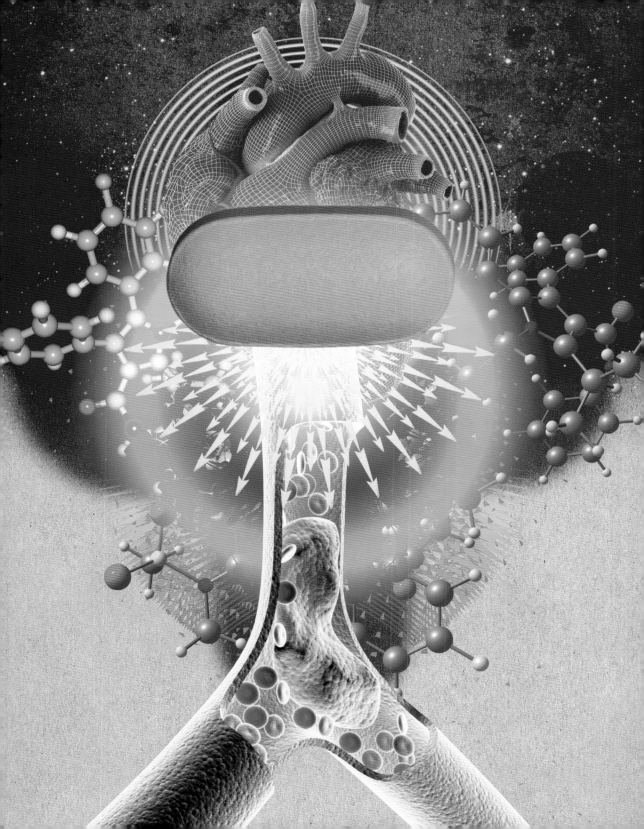

1836
Born in Whitechapel, East London, the second of 12 children

1854
Meets Emily Davies, co-founder of Girton College Cambridge, on a trip to visit friends in Gateshead

1859
Travels to London to meet Elizabeth Blackwell, the first woman in the USA to qualify as a doctor

1865
Passes exams and obtains a License of the Society of Apothecaries (LSA) allowing her to practice medicine

1866
Opens St. Mary's Dispensary for Women and Children to provide poor women with access to medical help from a female doctor

1870
Obtains medical degree from the University of Paris

1873
Becomes first female member of the British Medical Association

1874
Co-founds, with Sophia Jex-Blake, the London School of Medicine for Women

1908
Elected mayor of Aldeburgh, Suffolk, the first female mayor in Britain

1917
Dies at the age of 81

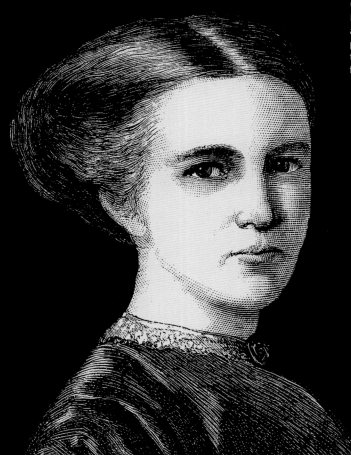

ELIZABETH GARRETT ANDERSON

Elizabeth Garrett Anderson was a true pioneer. Her unwavering determination to qualify as a doctor and be recognized as such by the then all-male medical profession of Victorian Britain paved the way for many other women to follow in her footsteps.

Garrett's life and career were shaped by two meetings she had as a young woman in the 1850s: first with Emily Davies, the campaigner for women's rights to university access, and second with Elizabeth Blackwell, the first female doctor in the USA. Davies and Blackwell both encouraged Garrett to pursue her goal of becoming a qualified physician. Elizabeth's father, although initially opposed to his daughter's entering the medical profession, also became a great supporter of her ambition.

Garrett's medical education began in 1860 as a surgery nurse at the Middlesex Hospital from where she received an honors certificate in chemistry and *materia medica*. After being rejected by several of the leading medical schools, she was finally admitted by the Society of Apothecaries whose charter did not enable them to exclude her on the basis of gender. She received her license to practice medicine from the society in 1865, scoring the highest marks of the seven candidates sitting the exam that day. Garrett would eventually receive her full medical degree from the University of Paris, five years later.

Now qualified, but unable to take up a position in a hospital because of her gender, Garrett opened her own practice in London. From small beginnings, the patient list grew, and on the strength of its success, she established St. Mary's Dispensary—an institution to enable poor women to obtain medical help from female physicians. In 1873, Garrett Anderson became the first female member of the British Medical Association. The following year, she co-founded the London School of Medicine for Women, the first medical school in Britain to train women. Garrett Anderson continued to work at the school for the rest of her career and served as its dean from 1883 until her retirement in 1902.

No less active in retirement than in her career, Garrett Anderson continued to campaign for women's suffrage and in 1908 was elected the mayor of Aldeburgh, Suffolk—the first female mayor in Britain. A year after her death, the New Hospital for Women (which had developed from St. Mary's Dispensary) was renamed the Elizabeth Garrett Anderson Hospital in her honor.

Philip Cox

PROTON PUMP INHIBITORS (PPIs)

Proton pump inhibitors are the most potent inhibitors of gastric acid production. Since their development in the 1990s, there has been a 1,000 percent increase in their usage and up to one in three adults will take a PPI at least once each year. The common indications for PPIs include gastro-oesophageal reflux disease, treatment of peptic ulcers, both in the stomach and the duodenum, and the eradication of *Helicobacter pylori* (the bacteria implicated in the cause of peptic ulceration and gastric cancer). They can also be used to prevent the gastrointestinal complications of taking non-steroidal anti-inflammatory medications, such as aspirin or ibuprofen. There are five forms of the medication: omeprazole, lansoprazole, pantoprazole, rabeprazole, and esomeprazole, each one of which has slightly different pharmacology. This affects not only their onset of action, but also their potency and metabolism. PPIs are considered to be safe, but because of their wide usage a few individuals will experience significant side effects. These include fractures, pneumonia, gastrointestinal infections, vitamin and mineral deficiencies, and kidney problems. Usually patients are initially treated with a short course of PPIs, but if their symptoms persist they should be referred for an endoscopic examination of their upper gastrointestinal tract before long-term use.

3-SECOND DOSE
Proton pump inhibitors are a class of drugs that are potent inhibitors of gastric acid secretion and are used to treat a range of acid-related upper gastrointestinal disorders.

3-MINUTE TREATMENT
Many patients who are commenced on PPIs will take them long term and the recommendations to their family doctors are that these patients should take the minimum dose that controls their symptoms. In the treatment of *Helicobacter pylori*, PPIs are combined with two antibiotics. The effectiveness of the treatment is usually confirmed with a urea breath test.

RELATED ENTRY
See also
CANCER
page 106

3-SECOND BIOGRAPHY
BARRY MARSHALL
1951–
Australian physician and professor of clinical microbiology at the University of Western Australia, who was the first to link *Helicobacter pylori* with peptic ulcers; in 2005 he was awarded the Nobel Prize for this discovery

EXPERT
Martin Veysey

PPIs inhibit the secretion of gastric acids in the stomach. They are widely used to treat many gastrointestinal disorders and to prevent side effects from other drugs.

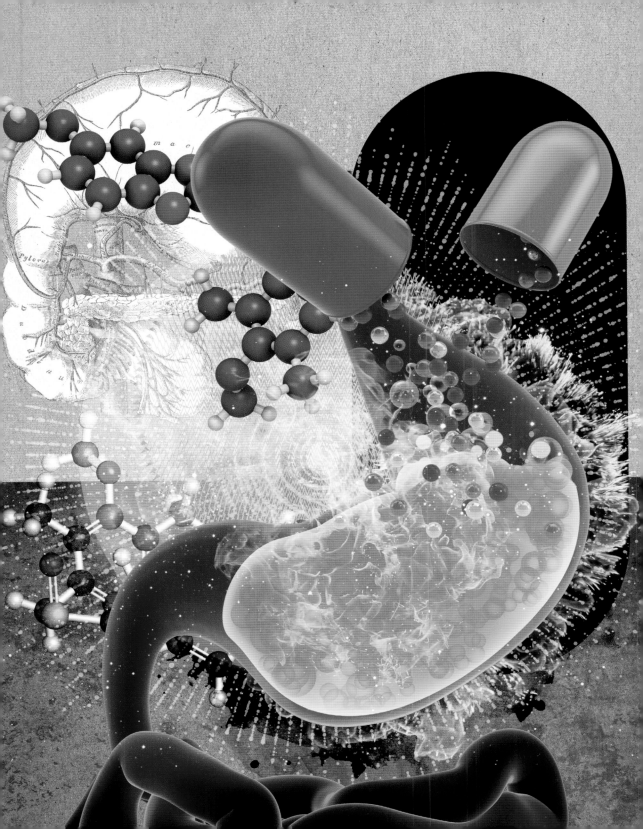

ANTICOAGULANTS

Normally in the human body

there is a fine balance between clot formation and destruction. This is controlled by a complex interaction between components of the blood, blood vessels, and the clotting cascade. The clotting cascade is a series of chemical reactions leading to clot formation. Some of these reactions are dependent on vitamin K. Factor X and thrombin are key chemicals in the cascade and are also targets for anticoagulant drugs. There are four main types of anticoagulant. Three can be administered orally, including warfarin (vitamin K antagonist), dabigatran (thrombin inhibitor), rivaroxaban, and apixaban (Factor X inhibitors). Heparin (inhibits thrombin and Factor X) must be given either intravenously or subcutaneously. Anticoagulants can be used to treat blood clots, such as deep vein thrombosis and pulmonary embolus, or to prevent clots from forming in high-risk individuals. Patients with an irregular heartbeat or heart valve replacements, surgical patients, and those with either a family history or personal history of clots, are all at increased risk. The main side-effect of anticoagulants is an increased risk of bleeding. This manifests as excessive nose bleeds and bleeding gums, but can be more serious. The effects of warfarin can be corrected by giving vitamin K or fresh frozen plasma. There is a specific antidote for heparin, but the effects of newer oral anticoagulants are not easily reversed.

3-SECOND DOSE

Anticoagulants are a group of medications, administered both orally and parenterally (by injection), that are used to prevent and treat blood clots.

3-MINUTE TREATMENT

Patients on warfarin and heparin will have its effects monitored by blood tests that assess the clotting cascade. The newer oral anticoagulants (apixaban, dabigatran, and rivaroxaban) do not require regular monitoring. A tendency to form clots is called thrombophilia. One of the commonest forms of familial thrombophilia is called Factor V Leiden and occurs in 5 percent of white Americans. Up to 30 percent of patients presenting with a deep vein thrombosis will have this condition.

RELATED ENTRY

See also
VASCULAR DISEASE
page 98

3-SECOND BIOGRAPHY

KARL LINK
1901–78
American biochemist who discovered the hemorrhagic factor produced in spoiled sweet clover hay that led to the development of warfarin

EXPERT

Martin Veysey

Anticoagulants are administered to patients at risk of blood clots. They work by interrupting the processes involved in the formation of clots.

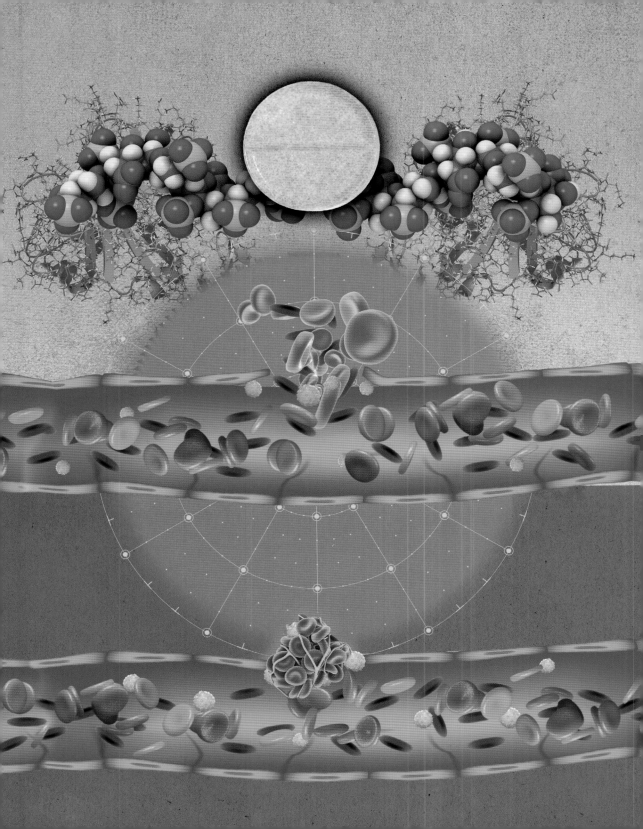

CANNABIS

3-SECOND DOSE
Cannabis is a restricted drug derived from the cannabis plant that is widely used as a relaxant and, more recently, for medicinal purposes.

3-MINUTE TREATMENT
About one in four of the adult population in the West admit to having tried cannabis at least once in their lifetime, and many of them use it regularly as a relaxant. Cannabis use causes an increased pulse rate, lowered blood pressure, and an increased appetite. It can lead to short-term memory loss and occasional psychiatric distress. There has been some concern about the link between cannabis use and long-term psychiatric conditions.

The oldest recorded use of the cannabis plant comes from China more than 4,000 years ago. The plant has many uses and originally spread globally when the Spanish imported it from Chile to use as a fiber. Cannabis grows wild in most parts of the world but is often cultivated commercially. As a drug, cannabis is legally restricted in most jurisdictions, and has a number of slang names including blow, Bob Hope, dope, ganga, hashish, marijuana, puff, skunk, and weed. Herbal cannabis contains more than 400 chemical compounds and over 60 cannabinoids. The most potent psychoactive cannabinoids are the tetrahydrocannabinols or THCs. Since the beginning of this century, regular cannabis users have been switching from cannabis resin to herbal variants of cannabis, leading to a significant increase in potency, with THC content of up to 15 percent. Cannabis is generally smoked in combination with tobacco, but can be eaten as cakes and cookies, or drunk as an extract. There are a number of medicinal uses of cannabis. Patients with neurological and musculoskeletal conditions may get symptomatic relief from pain and spasticity. Cannabis has also been used as an anti-nausea agent for patients receiving chemotherapy and to treat patients with increased pressure in their eyes (glaucoma).

RELATED ENTRIES
See also
TRADITIONAL CHINESE
MEDICINE (TCM)
page 24

CANCER TREATMENTS
page 72

3-SECOND BIOGRAPHY
SHEN NUNG
2737–2698 BCE
Chinese emperor and one of the fathers of traditional Chinese herbal medicine, who introduced cultivation of the cannabis plant to the Chinese people

EXPERT
Martin Veysey

Cannabis was one of the fundamental herbs used in traditional Chinese medicine. Its use in modern medicine is legally restricted; it is used for pain relief and as an anti-nausea agent.

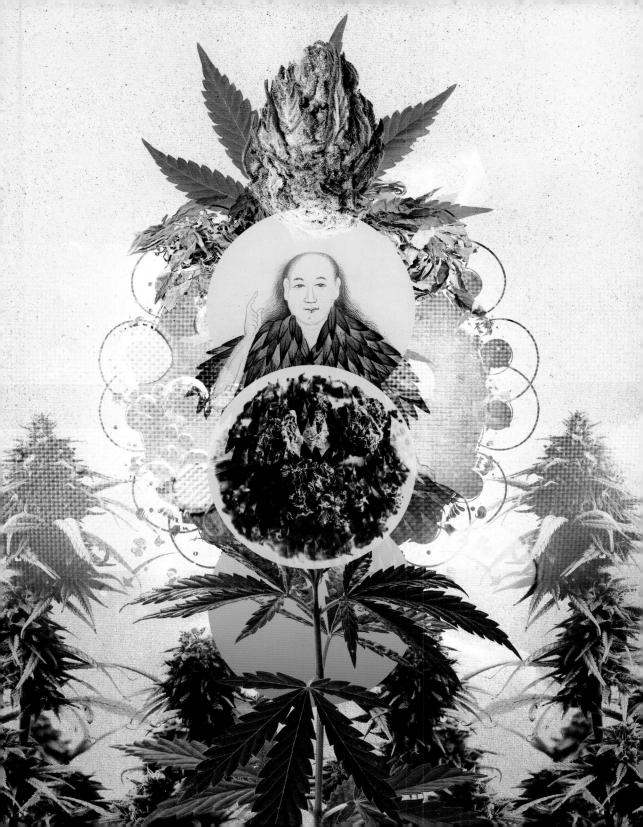

APPENDICES

RESOURCES

BOOKS

30-Second Anatomy
Gabrielle M. Finn
(Ivy Press, 2013)

Anatomy & Physiology For Dummies
Maggie Norris and Donna Rae Siegfried
(Wiley, 2011)

Blood and Guts: A Short History of Medicine
Roy Porter
(Penguin, 2003)

BMA New Guide to Medicine & Drugs
Dr Kevin M. O'Shaughnessy
(Chief medical editor)
(Dorling Kindersley, 2015)

The Cambridge History of Medicine
Roy Porter
(Cambridge University Press, 2011)

Crucial Interventions: An Illustrated Treatise on the Principles & Practice of Nineteenth-Century Surgery
Richard Barnett
(Thames & Hudson, 2015)

Gray's Anatomy (Classics Edition)
Henry Gray
(Barnes & Noble, 2011)

The Greatest Benefit to Mankind: A Medical History of Humanity
Roy Porter
(Fontana Press, 1999)

The History of Medicine: A Very Short Introduction
William Bynum
(Oxford University Press, 2008)

Kumar and Clark's Clinical Medicine
Parveen Kumar and Michael L. Clark
(Elsevier, 2016)

The Making of Mr Gray's Anatomy: Bodies, Books, Fortune, Fame
Ruth Richardson
(Oxford University Press, 2009)

Medical Terminology For Dummies
Beverley Henderson and Jennifer Lee Dorsey
(Wiley, 2015)

Oxford Handbook of Clinical Medicine
Murray Longmore, Ian Wilkinson,
Andrew Baldwin and Elizabeth Wallin
(Oxford University Press, 2014)

Virtual Anthropology: A Guide to a New Interdisciplinary Field
Gerhard W. Weber and Fred L. Bookstein
(Springer, 2011)

WEBSITES

American Journal of Medicine
amjmed.com

American Medical Association
ama-assn.org/ama

Canadian Institute for Health Information
cihi.ca/en

Centers For Disease Control and Prevention
cdc.gov

Health
health.com

Health Canada
hc-sc.gc.ca

Mayo Clinic
mayoclinic.org

MedBroadcast
medbroadcast.com

Medicine Net
medicinenet.com

Merriam Webster's Medical Dictionary
merriam-webster.com/medical

National Institutes of Health
nih.gov

Web Md
webmd.com

Web Md A–Z of Drugs and Medications
webmd.com/drugs

NOTES ON CONTRIBUTORS

EDITOR
Gabrielle M. Finn is Senior Lecturer in Medical Education at the Hull York Medical School. Gabrielle is an anatomist and educationalist who enjoys teaching a wide range of health care professionals. Her research interests include medical professionalism and anatomy pedagogy. Gabrielle is Education Chair for the Anatomical Society. Her PhD is in Medical Education.

CONTRIBUTORS
Philip Cox is a Lecturer in Physiology at the Hull York Medical School and the University of York. His research focus is the biomechanics and evolution of the masticatory system. Alongside his research and university teaching, Phil enjoys talking to the public about science and medicine, and has contributed to engagement events run by the National Science Learning Centre, the Prince's Teaching Institute, and the Cambridge Science Festival.

Laura Fitton is a Lecturer in Anatomy at the Hull York Medical School. She researches primate and human masticatory biomechanics applying various imaging modalities and virtual modeling techniques to the study of skull form and function. She teaches gross anatomy to medical students and virtual anatomy at postgraduate level.

Joanna Matthan is Lecturer at the School of Medical Education, Newcastle University, England, with a background in Medicine and English and a previous career in the corporate world. She predominantly teaches anatomy to medical and dental students but is also heavily involved in widening access to medicine and is passionate about teaching clinically relevant anatomy to postgraduate medical graduates training to be surgeons, anaesthetists, and radiologists. Her research interests range from anatomical themes to wider medical education ones.

Larissa Nelson is a Lecturer in the School of Biosciences at Cardiff University, Wales. She is an anatomist who is primarily involved in teaching medical and dental students. Her interests lie in the fields of anatomy, pedagogy, and medical education. Her PhD is in cartilage repair and she is currently completing a Master's in Education for the Health Professions. Larissa sits on the Anatomical Society Education Committee.

Martin Veysey is a gastroenterologist and clinical academic working within the School of Medicine and Public Health at the University of Newcastle in New South Wales, Australia. He trained in medicine at Guy's Hospital in the UK, and emigrated to Australia more than ten years ago. His interests include nutrition, genetics, medical education, and how to get the best possible outcomes for his patients.

INDEX

ACKNOWLEDGMENTS

PICTURE CREDITS
The publisher would like to thank the following for permission to reproduce copyright material:

Clipart.com: 38.
Getty Images/Popperfoto: 78.
Library of Congress, Washington DC: 15C, 51C, 51CR, 81TR, 100, 103TR, 119T & B (BG), 124, 129TR.
New York Public Library: 15CL, 63CR.
Science Photo Library/Martin Krzywinski: 37C.
Shutterstock: 15BR; 3D Vector: 23C; 3Dstock: 143T; A and N photography: 121TR; A-R-T: 137TR; Adike: 41BC; Adriaticfoto: 73T, 105T; Africa Studio: 21C; Aleksandr Kurganov: 151T (BG); Alex Mit: 109C; Alexandr III: 57C(BG); Alexilusmedica: 95BL, 103L, 139C; Alexonline: 35BR; Alfocome: 21TC; Algirdas Gelazius: 151T (BG); Alila Medical Media: 149C & B (main); Andrii Vodolazhskyi: 83CL & CR; Anton Gvozdikov: 31TC; Ase: 85BG; Attem: 57B; B Brown: 9BG, 77BG; Balein: 9TR, 77TR; Belekekin: 65BR; Blackboard1965: 18; Blackpixel: 121BL; Blamb: 41TR, 139C (overlay); Blue Planet Earth: 23BG; Boyan Dimitrov: 151C (L & R); Bruce Rolff: 95BG; Chirva: 21C; Chombosan: 61T; Creations: 43BC; Cristi180884: 75CR; Daivi: 141CR; Davydenko Yuliia: 141BR; Decade3d-anatomy online: 43TR, 71BL & BR, 83L & R, 147C; Designua: 45BC, 75C (L-R); Digital Storm: 35C, 35BL, 85TC; Dmitry Kalinovsky: 45T; Dny3d: 23T (BG); Dragana Gerasimoski: 33B (L to R); Dudarev Mikhail: 87BL; Duplass: 131C (body); Eder: 21BL; Everett Collection: 131TR; Everett Historical: 7C, 51TL, 71BR; Ewais: 2BL, 119BL; Extender_01: 107B (BG); Filmlandscape: 87BC; Flareimages: 117B; Foxterrier2005: 75C, 143CL, 143CR, 143B (BG); Frees: 51CL; Galushko Sergey: 43B (BG); Gen Epic Solutions: 107TL & BL; General-fmv: 55T & B; Grebcha: 9TR, 9CL, 9B, 77TR, 77CL, 77B; Gts: 23B; Herjua: 81C; Hjochen: 25TR; i3alda: 73C; Iodrakon: 131C (head); Jag_cz: 147C (BG); jannoon028: 123BG; Jezper: 73C; JFs Pic Factory: 35TR; JPC-Prod: 129TL (BG); Juan Gaertner: 95T & B, 95C, 97B (BG); Kalewa: 99T; Kateryna Kon: 9TC, 77CR, 83BG, 93BC, 103BL; Kathathep: 149C & B; Katsiuba Volha: 35BG; Kjpargeter: 65CR; Kletr: 93T; Kocakayaali: 41BR; Kondor83: 55T (BG); Koya979: 33TC; koya979: 33TR; Kreangkrai Indarodom: 141TC & CR; Kriangx1234: 123B; Kwangmoozaa: 75BR; Lenetstan: 127BR; LifetimeStock: 23CL; Lightspring: 99CL, CR & B; Linda Bucklin: 117C; MaluStudio: 73BG; marilyn barbone: 21BG; Marynchenko Oleksandr: 129C; Maximus256: 7BR; Maxx-Studio: 43BC; Maya2008: 137C; Meletios: 109C & B; Milles Studio: 151C; Molekuul_be: 9BR, 77BR, 81TL, 93BR, 97C, 105C, 137B, 139TR, 139CL, 147TL, 147CL, 149T, 149T (BG); Monkey Business Images: 2TR, 119TR, 121BL; Morphart Creation: 81BR; Mr. High Sky: 83B; Natykach Nataliia: 37C; Nav: 55 (Main), 65T, 73T; Nerthuz: 31C (L to R), 85C; Nixx Photography: 111TC & L; Nomad_Soul: 139BG; O2creationz: 141C; Oksana2010: 23CR; Oleksiy Mark: 129T (BG); Olga Zakharova: 111T; Ollyy: 87C; Ondrej83: 141TL; Onur Gunduz: 9C, 9BG, 77C, 77BG; Ostill: 121TL, 121C; OZMedia: 51BR; Paper Street Design: 65BG; Petarg: 103BG; Peteri: 93C; Petr Salinger: 81BR; Phovoir: 23T; Pogonici: 129B; Potapov Alexander: 121CR (BG); Poznyakov: 123L; Ppart: 129TR (BG); Praisaeng: 51TR; Pressmaster: 127T; Puwadol Jaturawutthichai: 53T & B, 109T (BG); Rafal S: 97TC; Raimundo79: 141B (BG); Raj Creationzs: 107C, 143BC; Ralf Neumann: 45BG; Ralwel: 105BL; Rawpixel.com: 37C (outer); Roberto Piras: 43TL' royaltystockphoto.com: 149C & B; Samuel Micut: 53C; Santibhavank P: 85L & R; Sarans: 139TL & BR; Sarayoot: 85 (BG); Science photo: 61B; Sciencepics: 33C, 43BC, 75TL; Sebastian Kaulitzki: 31L, 31C & BC, 31R, 33TL, 41L, 45BR, 83BG, 83BG, 95CL, 99C, 105TL & BR, 149BC; Sebastian Tomus: 61C; Sfam_photo: 123C (BG); ShaunWilkinson: 143C, 149TC; SkyPics Studio: 57C (BG); Sportpoint: 63C; Spwidoff: 127BL; Suthee Treewatanawong: 2TL, 119TL; Suwat Wongkham: 75TC; Syda Productions: 2CR, 119CR; Tefi: 95TR, 95BR; Terayut Janjaranuphab: 121BR; Thailoei92: 51BL; Timquo: 147TR; Toeytoey: 45BG, 93BG C & L; Tristan Tan: 25C; Tyler Olson: 123R; Valentyn Volkov: 31BG, 151BC; Vector FX: 99T & B (BG); Vereshchagin Dmitry: 131TL & BL; Ververidis Vasilis: 57T (BG); Vilor: 25BR; VirtualMaker: 53BG; Vladimir Arndt: 105B; Vladystock: 43C; Volodymyr Krasyuk: 75TL; Wavebreakmedia: 117T; Willyam Bradberry: 63BR; Wire_man: 111BC; Wk1003mike: 131BR; Xrender: 95CL (inner); YamabikaY: 151T.
U.S. National Library of Medicine: 87TL, 87CR.
Wellcome Library, London: 9TL, 15TL, 17TL, 17C (main), 17BC, 17BR, 21TL, 21TC, 25TL, 25BC, 57T, 58, 63TL, 63TR, 71TC, 71CL, 77TC, 85B, 87T (BG), 87BR, 97TL, 107CR, 107BG, 144, 151TC.

All reasonable efforts have been made to trace copyright holders and to obtain their permission for the use of copyright material. The publisher apologizes for any errors or omissions in the list above and will gratefully incorporate any corrections in future reprints if notified.